HEALTH AND BEAUTY

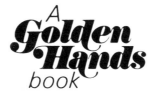

A *Golden Hands* book

Marshall Cavendish, London

Front Cover photograph by
Caroline Arber
Text by Sally Ann Voak
Edited by Sally Ann Voak
and Magda Gray
Co-ordinating Editors: Maggi
McCormick and Karen Harriman
Designed by Janet Sayer and
Andrzej Bielecki
Illustrated by Pat Ludlow
and Sue Richards
Preparation of food by Jane Oddie

Beauty
©Marshall Cavendish Ltd. 1974

Eating to be Healthy
©Marshall Cavendish Ltd. 1973

Photographs
John Aadrian: 1, 12, 13, 17, 37, 47, 48,
54, 60-61
Innoxa: 2
Elida: 5, 9, 27
Max Factor Ltd: 15, 41, 53
Transworld: 18, 31
Clairol Ltd: 27, 53, 64
Camera Press: 27
Ambré-Solaire Ltd: 28-29
Dudley Harris (Cutex Ltd): 33

Vanda Beauty Counselor: 44
Syndication International: 50, 57
Malcolm Scoular: 62
Camera Press: 122 (top), 128
Anthony Denny: 122 (bottom)
Paul Kemp: 83, 84, 85, 93, 95, 99, 100,
102, 103, 106, 111, 112, 113, 115, 118,
120, 127
Picture Library: 108
Spike Powell: 91
Malcolm Scoular: 65, 67, 73, 76, 79, 117
Transworld: 89
Patrick Ward: 75

We would like to thank the following:
Page 10-11: Make-up and brushes. Max
Factor Salon, London. Anello & Davide
Ltd, London. Bermans and Nathans
Ltd, London.
Page 15, 41: Make-up created by
Douglas Young, Chief Creative Make-
up Artist of Max Factor (London) Ltd.
Sweaters from a selection at Biba,
London.
Page 25: Hair settings by Harold
Leighton of Harrod's Hair Salon,
London.
Page 47: White nightdress
Page 48: Plaid rug and cushion from a
selection at John Lewis.

Published by Marshall Cavendish Publications Ltd.,
58 Old Compton Street,
London, W1V 5PA

©Marshall Cavendish Limited

This material first published by
Marshall Cavendish Ltd. in
Beauty and *Eating to be Healthy*

This volume first published in 1974
Printed in Great Britain by
Artisan Press Ltd.

ISBN 0 85685 071 3

This volume not to be sold in the U.S.A.
Canada and the Philippines

ABOUT THIS BOOK...

If you feel good you look good . . . and with the help of *All You Need to Know About Health and Beauty*, you'll look beautiful!

What is a beautiful woman? She may not have perfect features, nor a 36-24-36 figure, but she knows how to make the most of her looks. And she has a special quality—an inner glow—that makes her truly beautiful. That comes from good health.

The first half of this colour-packed book concentrates on beauty. After an honest assessment of your face and figure, you'll learn how to enhance your attributes—and disguise or correct your faults. The articles range from how to choose and use the cosmetics that are right for YOU, **even some** made from the foods you eat, to shaping up your figure and making the most of your bath-time. And you'll find one- and two-day beauty regimes as well as hints on how to look your best during the difficult months of pregnancy.

Although beauty may be only skin deep, health isn't. The second part of this book tells you, in straightforward language, why a well-balanced diet is important and what foods your body needs to keep you feeling healthy—and sexy too. You'll find a week-long Vitality Diet that's guaranteed to make you sparkle—and masses of delicious, sustaining, and inexpensive recipes for you and your family.

So make a start today. It's all here—all you need to know to keep yourself young, vibrant and beautiful.

CONTENTS

what is beauty?

It is the way you look, the way you move — above all, the way you feel. Nature can give you many of the separate parts of beauty — shining hair, healthy teeth, a neat figure — but the way in which they are combined and cared for is up to you.

In the following pages you can discover dozens of useful hints on how to keep your face and body healthy and attractive. You will find much more than the usual information about make-up and hairstyle. There are detailed sections here on such subjects as skin care, personal freshness, care of the mouth and teeth, healthy and attractive feet and hands.

Being beautiful means making the very most of your looks. It means knowing what physical drawbacks you have and what you can do to overcome them. This is, in fact, one of the most fascinating aspects of beauty care: seeing yourself clearly and enjoying what you see, because you can visualize all the possibilities for beauty in your face and body.

If your eyes are deep-set, or small or hidden by droopy lids, find out how to turn the problem into an asset.

If your elbows are rough, or your neck looks dingy, there is no need to feel that you have to hide them away. You need only refer to the clear, encouraging advice here. Then you will discover how easy it is to give back to any part of your body which may have been neglected a look of new-minted beauty.

If you know how to deal with any flaws in your own attractiveness, you are bound to feel greater self-confidence and that will add to your beauty. If you know that your whole body is sweet and fresh, that your hair-style suits your features, that your perfume is well-chosen, you will know, too, that you are looking and feeling your best.

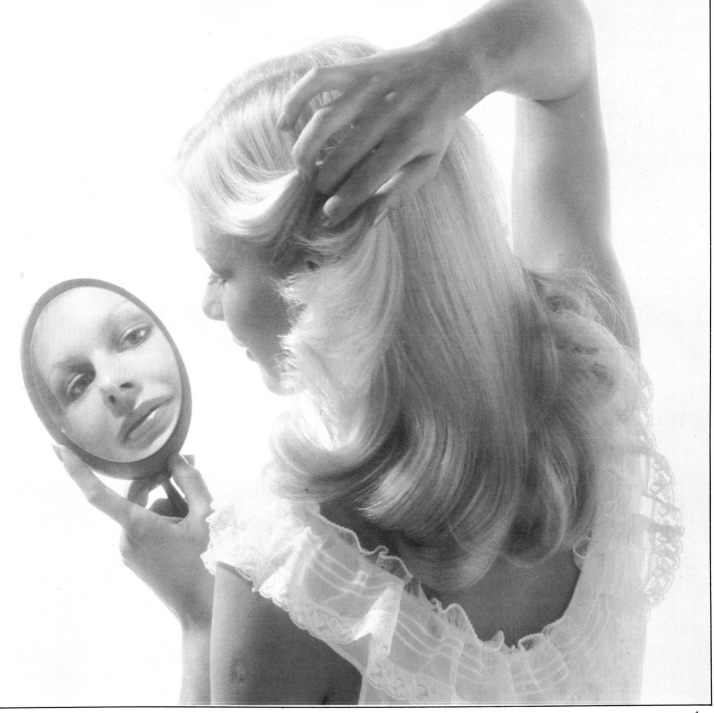

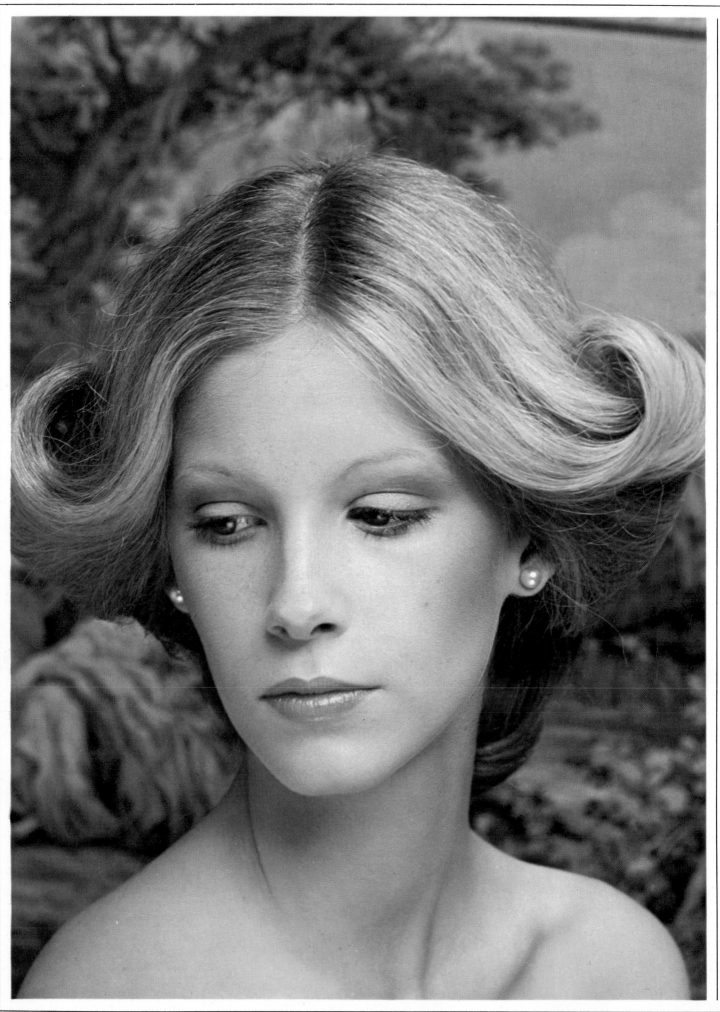

your face - learning to love it

The basis of the art of skilful make-up is honesty. The woman who looks good despite facial faults is the woman who knows what those faults are.

A careful assessment of face shape, of individual details such as hair-line, chin structure and the shape of the profile is the first essential step in using make-up successfully. The ideal make-up for you is the one that makes the best of your face — not necessarily the one that follows the fashion of the moment.

You need to take this close look at your face regularly. If your make-up hasn't changed much for some time, you are probably not making the most of your looks, for faces alter. The balance of your features now may mean that make-up which was exactly right for you even as little as a year ago is unsuitable now.

Remember, too, that in real life the face is rarely completely immobile. So other people hardly ever see the same face that you see when putting on make-up. Expressions of surprise, joy, attention, wonder and many more add the individuality which a perfect yet static mask of make-up does not have. While learning to know your face, learn to like it too. Even if it has faults, your face expresses a great deal about you, and if you do not like it, you can hardly expect that anyone else will, either!

Know your face

Take the hair back from your hairline with a bandeau, and sit in front of a mirror. Remove make-up. Now take a hand mirror and hold it in such a way that you can see the reflection of your face in the first mirror reflected in the second mirror. You are seeing your face, now, as others see it.

Check face-shape Forget individual features, and look at the outside con-

Play up a pale skin and pretty bone-structure with a porcelain-tinted foundation, eau-de-nil eye shadow and soft peach lipstick. Use a little amber blusher high on cheekbones

tour of your face. Is it round? Long? Square? Heart-shaped? Oval? If necessary, sketch in the outline on the mirror with an old lipstick to make sure.

Check profile Turn sideways to the mirror. Does the chin recede or jut forward? Is there a suspicion of a double chin? Is the nose prominent? Do the ears look large? Is the forehead domed?

Check features Are the eyes big small, deep-set or protruding? Are they round? Do they turn down at the outer corner? Are they wide apart or close together? The 'ideal' distance between them should equal the width of one eye. Is the nose turned up, aquiline, bulbous, small, large, crooked? Is the mouth small, large, well-defined, badly defined? Are both lips the same size or is the upper one smaller or larger than the lower? Are the ears neatly flat against the head, or do they stick out? Are the ear lobes small or large? Do the eyebrows match in size and shape?

Check balance The length of the face should be divided into three equal parts: hairline to bridge of nose, bridge of nose to tip, just under the nose to the point of the chin. Using this division as a guide, check whether forehead is high or low, chin long or short.

Now look carefully at the two halves of your face: they will not match exactly. One side may be wider at cheek or chin level. One eye is almost certainly bigger than the other. Lips may be fuller on one side, and the flare of one nostril broader than the other. These points are vital knowledge when you are applying make-up later, particularly when you are shading the contours of your face to obtain balance.

Preparing the canvas

After cleansing (with cream, liquid cleanser or soap and water — whichever is best for your skin) and toning, apply moisturizer all over your face and throat.

Now concentrate on skin and blemishes. Look for blemish scars, blotches,

exposed veins, dark circles under the eyes. (Using a dampened make-up sponge, and a covering stick make-up matched to your skin tone, cover these blemishes lightly.) Blemishes or pimples should be covered with a medicated disguise stick, slightly lighter in shade than surrounding skin tone, applied with a fine, clean, make-up brush. Allow a few seconds for this to dry, then apply a light liquid foundation. Use the sponge for this too, but wash it first.

If your skin is delicate, sensitive and prone to spots and blemishes, then choose a hypoallergenic (unperfumed) foundation and make sure the sponge is spotlessly clean.

Dab a little foundation on nose, cheeks, chin and forehead, then blend in carefully with light, outward strokes. Under the eyes, however, the strokes should be extra light — and in towards the nose. It is important for your foundation to blend with your skin tone exactly — and skin tone does alter occasionally. Always choose foundation carefully: try it on your face if possible, not on your wrist, which is very different from your face in tone and texture. You may find that it is a good idea to use several shades of the foundation which suits your skin. Blend the shades together in proportions that produce a lighter or darker colour according to your present skin tone. In summer, for instance, your skin may be quite golden, and become paler in autumn, very pale indeed in winter. Most women find that a beige-toned foundation is most flattering, because it will subdue any red or pink tints in the skin. A yellowish looking skin gains a look of health from a peachy-pink foundation.

For an olive complexion, choose a dark beige or tawny foundation. If your skin is dark brown or black, then look for the nearest blend you can find. Blend foundation lightly all over your face, including eyelids, throat and under chin. Make the layer as thin as possible around eyes and mouth: any lines there will be accentuated by a thick layer of foundation.

Balancing tricks

Look again into your mirror, this time with a face that is 'prepared'. Check over those shape and feature faults again. They are still there, and now is the time to start correcting them. Use two items for doing this: (A) a soft brownish-beige cake blusher with a soft, clean brush and; (B) a creamy-white cake highlighter, again with a soft, clean brush.

With just these two things, you will be able to remould your face. Start by concentrating on its contours.

Cheeks too wide Using A (the brown-beige blusher), brush a triangle of colour from cheekbone to chin level. Make the colour very soft and blend it in well. One cheek is probably chubbier than the other, so widen or lengthen the shaded triangle to even up the result, depending on where the chubbiness occurs.

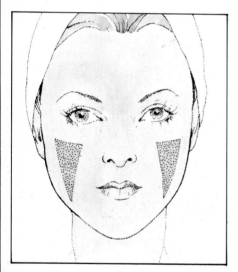

Chin too round Using A, shade a little colour on each side of your chin to diminish roundness. Using B, add a highlight to the centre of the chin to give a more pointed effect.

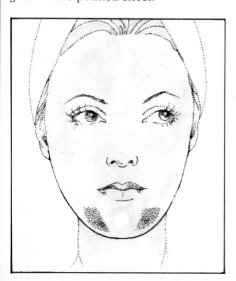

Forehead too broad Using A, add a very little colour to the sides of the forehead just above each brow-bone and blend well in.

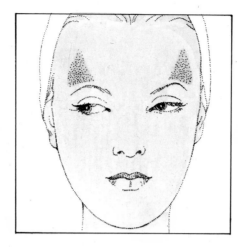

Nose too long Using A, brush a little colour very carefully over the tip of the nose and nostrils, blending it in very carefully with the main foundation and powder, so that you do not have any hard lines.

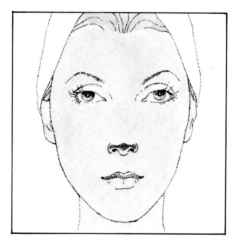

Jaw too broad Using A, make a small triangle of colour on each side of the jaw from mid-cheek down to chin-bone. Blend in carefully. Now study your separate features carefully.

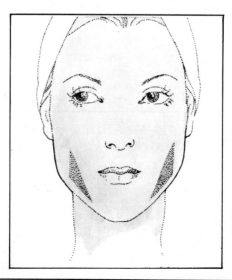

Nose too wide and flat Using B (the creamy-white highlighter), make a thin line down the centre of the nose (using an emery board or orange stick to keep the line straight). Now, using A, brush a little colour along the sides of the nose. Blend the two colours together where they touch, using a third soft brush.

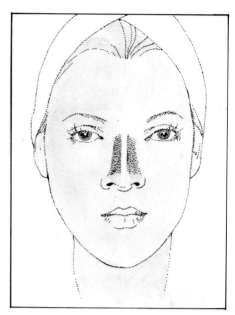

Eyes too close together Using B, add highlight to the space between the eyes and to the brow bone. This will have the effect of pushing the eyes outwards. Also check your brows (see point 6 under Making Beautiful Eyes), since cleverly shaped brows can often correct badly balanced eyes.

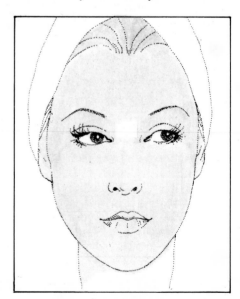

Once your 'balancing tricks' have been completed, powder over your entire face with a translucent loose powder on cotton wool [cotton]. Brush off the surplus with a soft brush. Your face is ready now for eye and lip make-up (in that order).

eyes - keep them sparkling

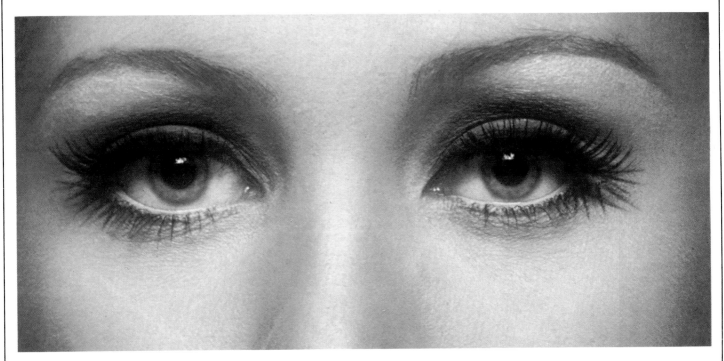

Like shiny hair and clear skin, bright eyes indicate glowing good health and vitality. If you become ill or run-down or if you just feel off-colour, your eyes will become dull and strained looking.

The first and most basic requirement for beautiful eyes is a good diet. The top vitamin for healthy eyes is Vitamin A, the one particularly associated with the ability to see in dim light. It is found in butter and margarine, oily fish like herrings, kippers, sardines, salmon and tuna. Its 'precursor' (a substance which can be quickly converted into Vitamin A by the body) is carotene — the orange pigment found in all orange and yellow fruits and vegetables, particularly carrots, apricots and turnips.

So, a diet which is rich in these foods will help to make eyes shine with health. For instance, you could try grated raw carrot on salads a few times a week, tuna fish for lunch occasionally, kippers for breakfast. As these foods also contain other nutrients vital for general good health, you will be benefitting your whole body, not just your eyes.

Tired, strained eyes Sleep is vital for bright, shining eyes. Without it they become bloodshot and tired-looking. Eight hours a night is a good rule. Use sleep like a bank, putting in extra hours when you have overdrawn. Watching TV for long periods or reading in bad light can also cause eye-strain. Check lighting at home and at work to make sure that it is adequate or perhaps even that it is not too bright. Some people find that fluorescent tube lighting can be very hard on their eyes. Many people need glasses (or need their existing lenses adjusted) without knowing it. If you know that you are getting enough sleep and yet your eyes look tired and you get headaches, consult your optician.

Smoking can make eyes dull-looking too; the nicotine can stain the whites of the eyes a dull, yellowish colour, just as it stains teeth and fingers. If you work in a smoky atmosphere, refresh your eyes daily with eye-drops recommended by your doctor or optician. Make sure, too, that you are able to get out of the smoke for a walk. One remedy for tired eyes, worth trying if you have to go out after a tiring day, is to lie down with a piece of cucumber over each eye. Remove your eye make-up first, of course. Then relax for a few minutes with your eyes closed. The cucumber is cooling and refreshing.

Puffy eyes Lack of sleep can make eyes look red and puffy. Never put heavy night creams, moisturizers or nourishing facial masques round the delicate eye area, for the oils they contain will stretch the fine skin and produce a puffy result. Beware, too, of letting astringent lotions, face packs or anti-spot lotions come into contact with this area: all of them contain drying ingredients which could cause wrinkling and aging of the skin.

Eye creams are always very light in texture. If you need to use an eye cream for dryness, then pat it in very sparingly with the pad of your forefinger, keeping the touch delicate and light. Puffy eyes can sometimes be helped if you cleanse your whole system by drinking eight glasses of water a day.

Dark circles under the eyes Acute fatigue or strain can cause this problem. If insomnia is the root of the trouble, try to relax before sleep by doing a few yoga exercises or by taking a brisk walk. If the insomnia persists, you should consult your doctor. Meanwhile, the dark circles can be disguised with a pale, light-textured foundation in liquid or cake form applied very lightly with a soft bristle brush or a moistened make-up sponge.

Crow's feet and laughter lines The skin under and surrounding the eyes is very delicate indeed, and sometimes tiny lines may even appear in very dry teenage skins. Although the lines, once formed, cannot be removed except by surgery, it is possible to delay the line-forming process by keeping the skin soft and supple. Never drag the skin when removing eye make-up. Always use a good eye make-up removing cream on cotton wool [cotton] — tissues are too rough for this operation. Baby oil is likely to lubricate the area too much, causing puffiness and probably stretching the skin, so it should be used sparingly. After removing make-up, pat in a very little eye oil or cream just under the lower lashes. There are also some eye creams which are protective and designed to be worn under make-up during the day. Do not worry about laughter lines: these can add to your beauty. A perfectly smooth face can be a very boring one.

Eye make-up allergies Most women experience some kind of eye make-up allergy trouble during their lives. Unfortunately, this can suddenly happen with a favourite mascara or shadow which has been perfectly satisfactory for years. If redness or itching start, you may have simple conjunctivitis or an irritation or abrasion caused by a foreign body in the eye. If the discomfort is not cleared up by eye drops prescribed by your doctor, you may be allergic to your eye make-up. Stop wearing it for a day or so. If the redness and itching disappear, replace your existing eye make-up with items from a non-perfumed hypoallergenic range. These are now available in lovely colours and textures, so you won't sacrifice any fashionableness.

Caring for your eyelashes Eyelashes drop out regularly and grow again, just like the hair on other parts of the body. However, they do tend to become sparse and brittle if they aren't well cared for. One of the biggest dangers is in not removing mascara properly. Do this with the utmost care, with several applications of the eye make-up removing cream. If your lashes are out of condition use a simple non-waterproof cake mascara with no thickening fibres. This is easier to remove and better for the eyes and you can still get a thick, soft effect by applying several layers and powdering the lashes between applications. Some waterproof mascaras need hard rubbing to remove them — bad for the skin under the eye and ruinous for the lashes. Beware, too,

of wearing false eye lashes (see below) too often and never mascara them so that they stick to your own eye lashes. You are bound to pull a few of the precious real lashes out when removing the false ones. It isn't worth it.

To help lashes grow long and lustrous, apply a very little almond oil to them every night. Make sure that the oil

cannot go into your eyes, however, and keep it well away from the skin below the eyes.

If you have very pale lashes it is worth considering dyeing the lashes darker to give a natural emphasis to your eyes with or without make-up. Have this done professionally: it is a very tricky job requiring a steady hand.

False eyelashes False eyelashes should be put on in the following way: hold the lashes in tweezers and apply a hairline of adhesive along the edge of the eyelash band only. Look downwards slightly into a swivel mirror on a stand, hold the lash band above eye level and bring down towards the lid. Place the mid-point of the lash band above the centre of the eye and press gently into position. Now press the whole base of the lash band into position right along the lid, using either the applicator provided in the pack or tweezers. Finally, massage the eyelid skin downwards. The white adhesive will become colourless as it dries. Blend false and real lashes together for a natural look using a dry eyebrow brush. To remove the lashes, take the outer corner of the lash band carefully between finger and thumb and gently pull away from the lid. Clean off the hairline strip of adhesive by simply pulling it off with tweezers. (Any stubborn adhesive should be removed with soap and water.)

False eyelashes can be curled by being wrapped round a pencil with a tissue and left overnight.

A new technique, now available at some beauty salons, fixes individual false lashes 'permanently' to the eyelids. However, the added lashes are shed after about two or three weeks — and they can sometimes drop out at embarassing moments.

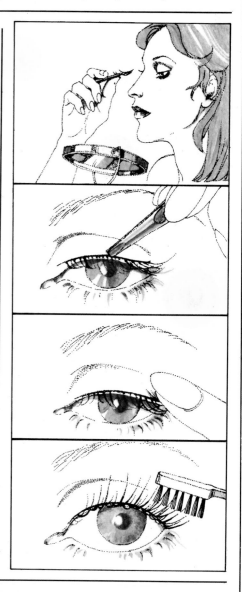

SIX SIMPLE EYE EXERCISES

When you are doing any close work — sewing, reading or typing — it's a good idea to break off occasionally to rest and relax your eyes with some simple exercises. Try these:

1 Look up and focus on an object at the other end of the room. Now, without moving your head, switch your gaze to an object which is close at hand. Focus on the two objects, alternately, 20 times each

2 Rotate your eyes clockwise: lift them up to the left, round to the right, down on the right, then back to the left again. Repeat 10 times. Rest.

Now rotate anti-clockwise. Repeat 10 times. Rest

3 Raise your eyes diagonally leftwards to the ceiling, then lower them to the floor. Repeat 10 times. Repeat the exercise a further 10 times, raising your eyes diagonally rightwards

4 Cup your hands over your eyes and stare into the blackness for a few moments

5 Close your eyes, count two, then open them again, count two, then close them. Repeat 20 times

6 Look up and blink rapidly for a count of 20. Rest. Look downwards and repeat blinking

making beautiful eyes

One of the most exciting developments in make-up in recent years has been the interest in eye beauty products. A vast quantity of these are now available to choose from, and that can sometimes be confusing. Most women develop a preference for one type of mascara — cake, spiral, cream or comb-on. But when they are choosing eye shadow, they find that the range is so vast that it is hard to make a selection. Here's a simple rule: if you want to try a completely new type of shadow — say, a pearly cream one instead of your usual powder, then buy one of the cheaper ranges. If the new type is a mistake, it won't be such a costly one, and if it's a success, you can always choose a more expensive pearly cream shadow in a subtler colour next time.

Shadow — whether it's a cream (in a tube), stick, powder or greasy gloss (in a pot) — should always be applied with a brush. A brush gives you more control over application and produces a more accurate, lasting effect. Don't be afraid to blend colours to produce a subtler shade: most models are skilled at producing their 'own' cosmetics in this way. Use a little moisturizing cream to help mix the two products smoothly. Here is a step-by-step guide to a successful eye make-up:

Putting on eye make-up

1 Make sure foundation covers the eyelids completely, then powder over with translucent loose powder to give a matte surface to work on. If your eyelids tend to be pink and blotchy, cover them completely with a beige cream shadow, then powder and work on top of this camouflage.

If eyelids are crepey in texture, do not use foundation under eye make-up. Simply apply moisturizer and loose powder, and always use a powder eye shadow. Creamy or glossy shadows will tend to form creases on an uneven surface. The lighter the eye make-up the better. A thick layer may cake and crack.

2 Adjust your mirror so that you are looking slightly downwards into it. A small mirror on a stand on top of your dressing table is best, particularly if it has a magnifying side. Make sure that you can rest your elbows comfortably on the table-top as you work, for this is the best way to keep your hands really steady.

3 What you will need Select the items you intend to use. Three blending or toning shadows: one for the lid, one for the crease of the eye, one for the brow bone. A wedge-shaped brush for each eye shadow. Eye brow pencil: very sharp. Tweezers to pluck out any stray brows (eye brow shaping is a separate job: see point 6 below). Mascara and brush. Eyeliner and brush.

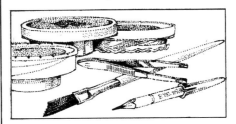

4 Eye shadow Apply lid shadow first in light strokes, then crease shadow and finally the shadow on the brow bone. See the diagrams below under Placing and Shape for tricks on how to improve your eye shape.

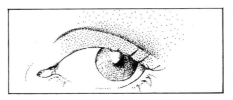

5 Mascara Now apply mascara very carefully — in upward strokes on top lashes and downward strokes on the bottom ones. Apply one coat, allow it to dry, then apply a second coat. For a thick, soft look without fibres (which can irritate the eyes and clog lashes), powder between each coat. Finally, separate the lashes with a dry brush for a natural, feathery look.

6 Eye brow pencil Apply pencil to brows, following the natural curve in very light feathery strokes, not a hard line. As you work, tweeze away any hairs which spoil the line, but below the brow only. Brush brows gently to give a smooth line and to soften the

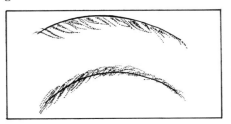

pencil marks. For an even softer effect, first brush the brows downwards, then draw in brow shape with soft strokes and finally brush brow hairs upwards again to cover the line.

7 Eyeliner If you intend to use eyeliner, apply it now. A dark, heavy line is definitely unflattering. Choose a shade which is close to that of the shadow on your lid and make a soft, smudgy line, not a hard one. To give the eyes an almond shape, apply the line from the centre of the lid, very

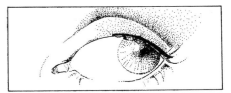

close to the lashes, to the outer corner of the eye, thickening it slightly on the way. Apply a little eye shadow on top of the line to make it even softer and more subtle.

Removing eye make-up

Always use a product which is gentle and specially formulated for this purpose. Baby oil is fine if used very sparingly indeed and so long as care is taken not to allow the oil to trickle into the corners of the eyes. Proceed like this:

1 Remove false eye lashes if worn (see Caring for your Eye Lashes)

2 Apply a little eye make-up remover to a pad of cotton wool [cotton] — dampened if you find this easier

3 Now close one eye and wipe the cotton wool [cotton] gently from the outer corner in towards the nose. Repeat several times, then open eye. Using a fresh pad of cotton wool [cotton], wipe inwards under the lower lashes.

Eye make-up allergies

Occasionally, a product may produce an allergy. Check that eye make-up brushes and eyeliner brushes are all scrupulously clean. Never use saliva as a solvent. If a product makes eyes sore or watery, do not persist with it. There are several good hypoallergenic ranges on the market which use no perfume in their eye make-up formulae — it is the perfume which is very often responsible for an allergic reaction in some users. Manufacturers are usually quite willing to test products if a complaint is made. If soreness persists after you cease using the product, check with your doctor immediately.

Placing and shape

Skilful make-up can disguise problems.
Eyes too close together Widen the space between your brows first by careful plucking. Make a 'wing' of shadow from the centre of the lids upwards and outwards towards the outer points of the brow. Add a little liner to the outside edge of the lid only and concentrate mascara on the outside lashes. You can put on an extra coat or two to build up a little extra density.

Eyes too protruding If the lids are prominent, giving a hooded effect to the eyes, use a dark, muted shadow all over them to make them recede. Smooth a lighter shadow from the socket to the brows to bring this area forward slightly.

Eyes too deep-set Reverse the procedure for protruding eyes, applying a lighter shadow to lids, and a darker one from the socket crease to the brows. You will find that your eyes seem to come forward quite noticeably. Put on plenty of mascara, lightly applied, or use feathery false lashes to give extra size and prominence to your eyes.

Eyes too wide apart Add a little extra shadow matching the shadow on the eye lids to each side of the bridge of your nose to make the space between the eyes look narrower. If brows grow wide apart, bring them closer together with a few strokes of pencil at the inner corners, but be sure to do this very subtly, drawing perhaps just three or four 'false hairs'.

Eyes too droopy 'Bloodhound' eyes can be made less droopy if you concentrate eye make-up on the centres of the eyes — leaving the outer corners untouched. Let shadow curve upwards and outwards towards the brows to 'lift' the eyes. If your brows also droop downwards at the ends, pluck away the hairs from underneath and pencil in extra ones on top to raise the brow.

Eyes too round Pluck eyebrows into an angular shape, not a round arch. Give eyes an almond look by starting eyeliner halfway between the centre of the lid and the outer corner, gradually thickening the line towards the end. Blend shadow softly from the centre of the lid, deepening the colour and concentration at the outer edge and extending it a little way beyond the outer corner of the eye.

Eyes too narrow Give a rounded effect by using shadow under the bottom lashes as well as on top of the lid. Make special use of mascara on bottom lashes. Shape eye shadow in an upward curve from the centre of the upper lid towards the brow.

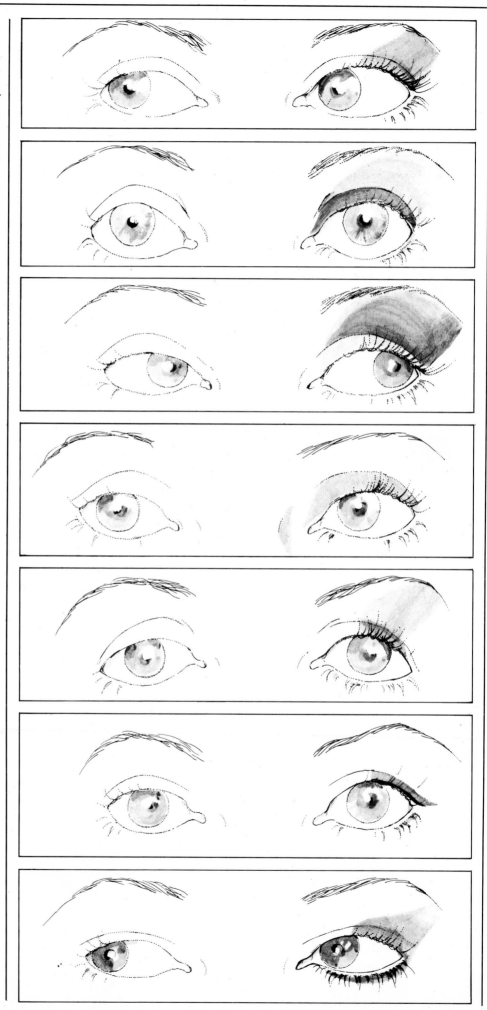

lips -

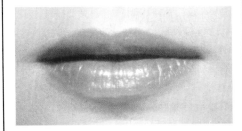

shape & colour

In the last ten years or so, glossers, see-through lipsticks, creamier formulae and unusual colours have appeared to broaden the whole idea of lip make-up. And a new, flattering lip colour is still one of the best, most inexpensive morale boosters. In fact, latching on quickly to new lipstick shades is a good way to stay abreast of fashion.

Testing lip colour To test lip colour in a shop, apply the tester stick to the tip of your finger and hold this close to your mouth. Look at it in relation to skin colouring, eyes, hair. Next, think of it in relation to the clothes which you will be wearing with it.

Applying lip colour This needs great care if the result is to be flattering and long lasting.

Here is a step-by-step guide:

1 Examine the texture of your lips first. If they are hard and cracked looking, soften with lip balm or moisturizer. Apply a thin film of creamy foundation over the whole of the lip area and powder lightly. The foundation can be the one you normally use on your face if the texture is light and greasy enough to cover lips without drying the delicate lip skin. If not, use an extra greasy foundation or tinted moisturizer bought specially for the purpose.

2 Adjust your mirror height carefully, so that you are looking slightly downwards at your mouth, with your elbows resting neatly and comfortably on the table. Use the magnifying side of the mirror, if it has one, for application, the plain side to check the effect as you go along

3 Assemble cosmetics and equipment: lipstick(s) or lip colour in a pot, lip brush, glosser, brush, tissues

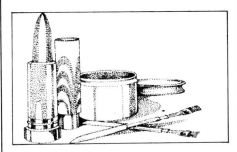

4 First draw in the outline of your lips with a well-filled brush (see the sketches for tricks to disguise faults in lip shape)

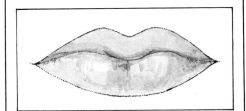

5 Now fill in the colour, following the outline very carefully. You may find that using two colours — separately or blended — gives a more interesting effect. Experiment carefully

6 If lip colour tends to 'smudge' into skin surrounding the mouth, blot the colour with a tissue and re-apply carefully

7 Apply clear or toning lip gloss all over the mouth for a shiny look. When retouching lipstick in public, it is easier and more elegant to use the stick direct. However, if you have used a brush to draw a firm outline at the beginning of the day, you will find that a simple 'filling in' is all that is necessary — the outline will still be there.

Structural improvements

Lips too thin Cheat a little by extending the outer line a little above your top lip, and below your bottom lip, and well into the corners of your mouth. A paler lip colour in the centre of the lips, with a darker one on the outside gives the impression of a fuller, more generous mouth.

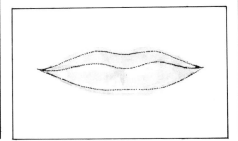

Lips too thick Reverse the process just described: drawing the outer line a little way inside the natural contours of your mouth. Use a darker shade on the centre of the mouth, a slightly lighter one outside to make the mouth look smaller.

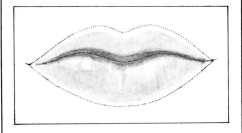

Lips too droopy Make the lip line tilt upwards at the corners of your mouth. (Smiling is a good natural treatment for this fault!)

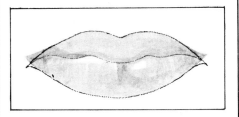

Lips uneven Most women have slightly uneven lips: the top lip may be thin, the lower lip thick — or one side of the lip may be shaped quite differently from the other. Observe your mouth closely and correct these faults as you draw the all-important outline.

Blueish lips If lips are blue looking, a yellow tinted lipstick worn under a normal colour will help. Beware of blueish-reds, hot pinks, mauvy shades.

Lipsticks that darken Lipsticks which turn darker after being worn for some time or leave an ugly stain on the mouth are most commonly those containing eosin — the chemical fixative which gives lipstick its lasting power. If you have dry lips, or lips which tend to look stained and cracked, choose a greasy formula lipstick without eosin. This will need reapplication frequently, but the colour will remain true.

Lip gloss Full, well-defined lips often look good with tinted lip gloss instead of lipstick. If your complexion is florid or mauve toned, then choose a brownish or tawny lipstick shade (and apply a covering foundation to tone down the hot colour of your skin.)

Lips in need of special care Dryness, cracking and soreness of the lips can sometimes be aggravated or even caused by the perfume in lipstick. Look for a hypoallergenic brand containing no perfume.

the well-equipped dressing table

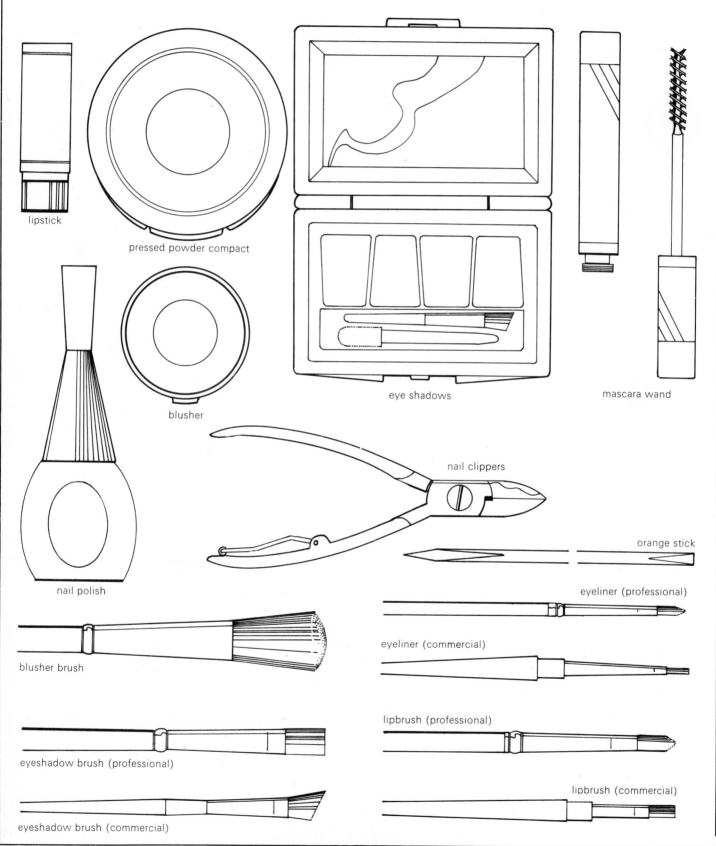

lipstick

pressed powder compact

eye shadows

mascara wand

blusher

nail clippers

nail polish

orange stick

eyeliner (professional)

blusher brush

eyeliner (commercial)

lipbrush (professional)

eyeshadow brush (professional)

eyeshadow brush (commercial)

lipbrush (commercial)

Skin care equipment

Cleanser
Cream or liquid. Once you find the type which suits your skin it's more economical to buy large sizes. Use generously.

Toner
Large size again. Rosewater is a good, inexpensive toner for normal to dry skins.

Moisturizer
Should be non-greasy, readily absorbed.

Night cream
Even creams for very dry skins are now quickly absorbed—there's no need to go to bed with a greasy face!

Under-eye cream or oil
A small pot lasts ages, since it is always applied very sparingly. Use the pads of your second finger and a tight touch.

Facial masks
Buy in sachet form until you find the best one for your skin—then buy a tube or jar.

Make-up

Foundation
Liquid, cream, stick or block (use with water and a sponge). Look for light texture—heavy foundations look artificial.

Blemish stick
Medicated cover-stick colour-toned to blend with your skin. Always apply with a clean brush, not straight from the stick.

Loose powder
A translucent shade is best since one colour will go over all skin-tones and most people's colouring varies quite noticeably according to weather, health, age, etc.

Solid compact
For touching up make-up only. Pressed powder tends to clog the skin and doesn't last as long as the loose kind. If you prefer, use a compact containing loose powder.

Blusher
Stick, powder, cream or gel.

Highlighter
Cream or powder in white or cream with a frosted look. Some manufacturers make sets containing blusher and highlighter together.

Eye shadow
Cream, powder, solid block (to use with water), liquid or gel. Have a good selection to go with mood, clothes, different make-up.

Eye liner
Solid or liquid (sometimes in a wand).

Mascara
Block or automatic, with or without thickening fibres.

False eyelashes
Keep them in the box, or curled around a pencil or make-up brush.

Lipsticks
Traditional lipstick-shaped container, in pot form or as a colour wand with brush included. The latter can be messy, however.

Lip gloss
Clear to go over lipstick or in soft colours to wear alone. Tiny pot lasts a long time.

Make-up brushes and equipment

Soft tissues
The softest you can find—harsh tissues drag delicate face skin. If you remove eye make-up with tissues instead of cotton wool [cotton], really soft ones are vital.

Cotton wool [Absorbent cotton]
Top quality, not surgical. Hard fibres may drag your skin and will certainly make jobs like removing old nail polish much more messy. Look for the cosmetic cotton wool [cotton] which is usually sold in 'balls' or 'pads'

Make-up sponges
Keep about 6, use a clean one every time. Made from very soft, flesh-coloured plastic foam, they are available from cosmetic counters and theatrical shops.

Blusher brush
A 'fat', very soft brush is necessary. The short, hard brushes supplied in blusher compacts are unsuitable for subtle effects.

Eye shadow brush
Straight-edged $\frac{1}{4}$-inch wide for applying browbone and eyelid shadow. It's easier to see what you are doing if the handle is long.

Fine eyeliner brush
Again, a long-handled theatrical brush is easiest to use.

Wedge-shaped eye shadow brush
For applying shadow in the eye socket. Commercial kinds have a short handle.

Lipbrush
Soft, pointed brush (choose soft sable if you can) with a long handle.

Covered lipbrush for handbag
It isn't practical to carry around a long-handled make-up brush with you, so tuck a covered lipbrush into the make-up bag in your handbag for touching up during the day.

Covered eyeliner brush for handbag
This, too, is easier to carry about than a long-handled brush.

Velours powder puffs
Easier to use than sponge or fluffy powder puffs. Keep several, wash them regularly.

Cotton buds
Available at the baby goods counter at your chemist [drugstore]. Invaluable for removing stray dark splodges of make-up without messing up the whole effect. Also good for cleansing one specific area such as your eyes without removing the rest of your make-up.

Manicure

Polish remover
Look for a gentle, oily type which is kind to nails. The bigger the bottle, the more economical your buy. Store well away from heat.

Cuticle remover
Usually in brush and bottle form.

Cuticle cream
A small pot or jar.

Nail clippers
Should be sharp!

Nail scissors
Sharp, with fine curved point for awkward corners.

Emery boards
Rough side for trimming, the fine one for smoothing rough edges. Keep a good stock and discard when worn. More effective than a metal file and less damaging to nails.

Orange sticks
The pointed end is for removing dirt and old polish trapped under the nail, the wedge-shaped end for gently easing back cuticles.

Base coat
Usually a pale pink nail polish — really does help the top coat to last longer.

Top-coat nail polish
Do not keep too many colours on the go at the same time since most varnishes tend to solidify once open. Keep a bottle of varnish solvent for thinning in emergencies.

Hair setting equipment

Hair grips and pins
Non-scratchy.

Mesh rollers
In various sizes. The type favoured by hairdressers wrap plastic mesh around wire. Spikes and brushes in rollers will tangle and pull long hair, although a small brush roller may be the best choice for holding very short hair.

Hair dryer
Hooded, salon-type or blower.

Hair net
Setting lotion
Shampoo
The mildest kind you can find.

Conditioner
Large soft hairbrush
Natural bristle if possible.

Large-tooth comb
Useful for untangling hair after washing.

Tail comb
For hair-setting.

Sticky tape
For setting small side and back curls.

Hairspray
Bathtime equipment
Bath mitt
Made from rough linen or towelling.

Loofah or back brush
Non-scratchy.

Nail clippers and pumice stone
Bath oil and bubble bath
Talc and body lotion
De-fuzzing equipment
Ladies' razor or electric shaver
Depilation cream and wooden spatula
Micellaneous
Make-up purse for handbag
Large sponge bag for travelling
Plastic jars
Heated rollers
Sun tan lotion
Perfumes

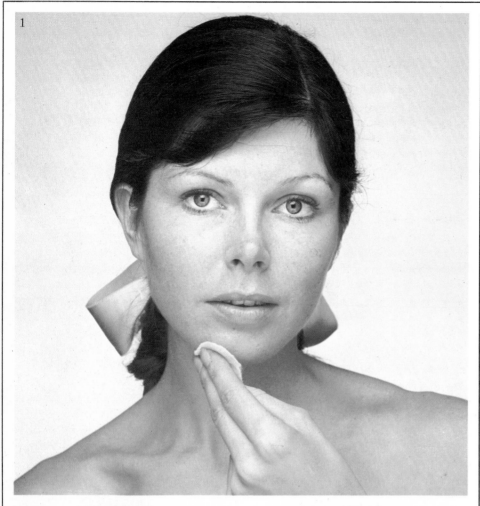

making up

The way to apply make-up is illustrated in two stages. The first gives a complete daytime face. Allow about 15 minutes for all six steps. The second stage transforms the basic daytime make-up into an evening look in three extra steps. If your eyes look tired or bloodshot, refresh them with eye-drops before putting on the eye make-up.

Daytime make-up

1 Deep cleanse with cream or liquid cleanser, then tone with skin freshener or astringent, especially down the centre panel—forehead, nose, and chin.
2 Apply moisturizer with fingertips, using light, outward, circular movements. Next apply foundation and powder. Press the powder into the skin in 'rolling' movements (see the photograph above) using a flat velours puff.
3 Brush brows into a neat, slightly curved line. Pluck out any straggly hairs. Darken the line and extend it if necessary with a well-sharpened eye pencil applied in feathery strokes. Next, use a creamy beige shadow over the entire eyelid area, smoothing the shadow up to the brows. Apply brownish-beige powder shadow to the lid. Apply darker brown powder shadow into the eye crease and creamy highlighter just under the brow. It is important to blend the colours together softly so that they merge into one another. Use a light touch and a wedge-shaped eye shadow brush.
4 Complete the eye make-up with a fine line of brown eyeliner very close to the upper lashes from the centre to the outside corner. Repeat under the lower lashes. Finally, brush on brownish-black mascara, using light upwards strokes on upper lashes, and downward strokes on lower lashes. It is important to apply the mascara to lower lashes to give a finished look to the eye.
5 Apply triangle of soft brown frosted blusher. Simply fluff on the blusher with a large brush. The triangle should stretch from just under the cheekbone, along the jawbone to a point level with the corner of the mouth.
6 Use a lip-brush to define outline. Fill in with brush or from the stick.
Brush out hair to complete your daytime look.

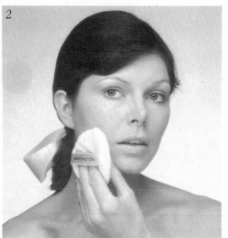

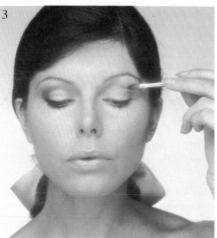

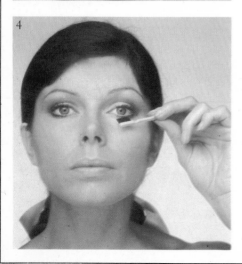

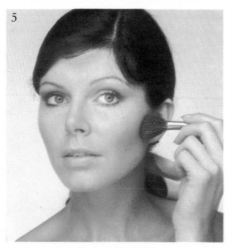

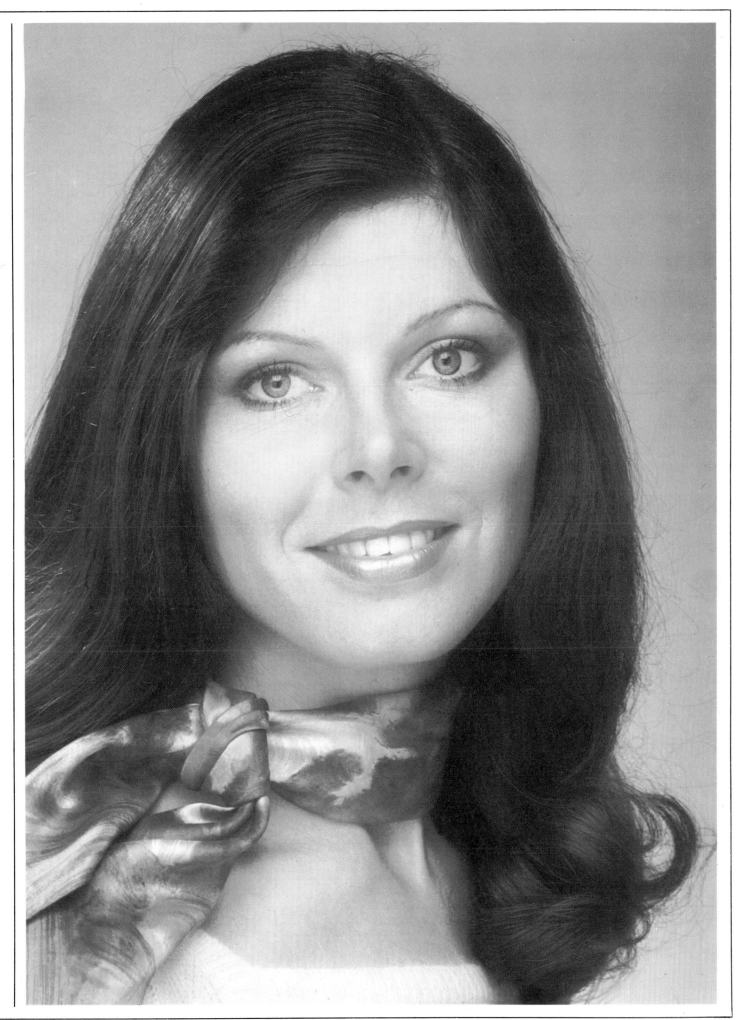

making up after six

Evening make-up

1 Remove lipstick with cleanser and tissues. Remove eyelid colour and browbone highlighter very gently with cotton buds. There is no need to remove foundation, blusher or mascara. Darken eyebrows slightly. Add a deep blue powder shadow to lids, a greyish-brown shadow in the eye crease. Finally add a frosted white highlighter to the brow bone. To give the shiny look shown in the picture, add a line of highlighter a $\frac{1}{4}$ inch wide down the centre of each lid *over* the deep blue shadow.

2 Redefine lip line with a brush and fill in with a deeper, warmer lip colour. Top with glosser for a shiny look.

3 Add warmth to cheekbones with a touch of peachy blusher just above the daytime triangle of brownish blusher.

A rapid switch from daytime to evening make-up is possible with just a few well-planned colour and tone changes

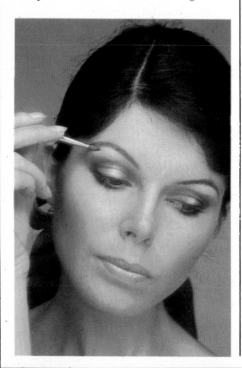

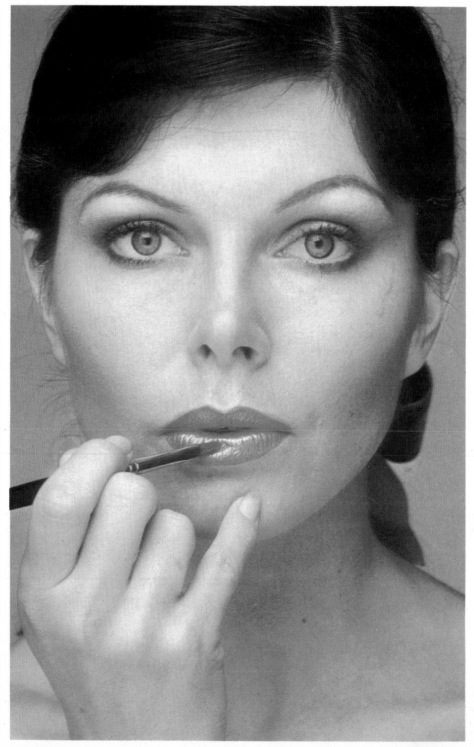

14

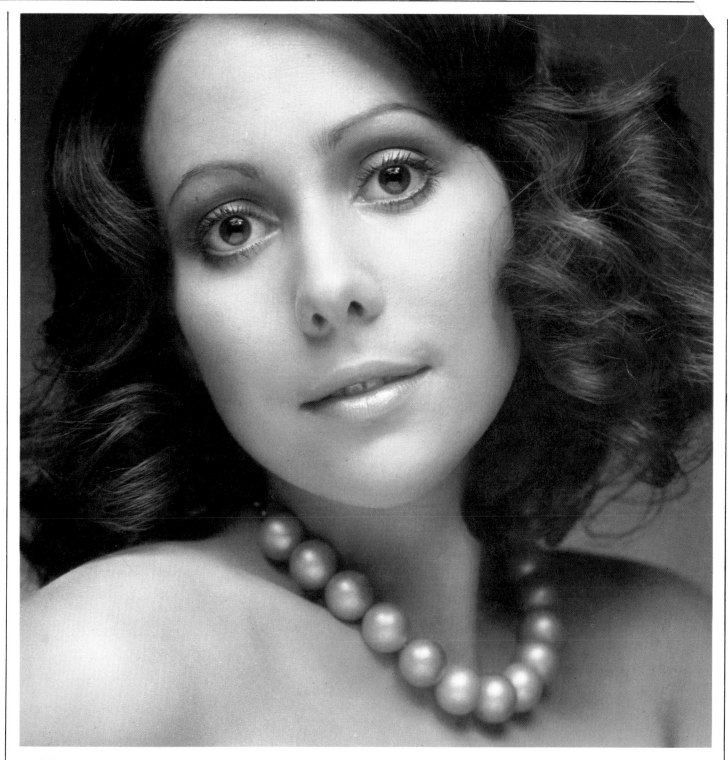

Quick Change—
Day-into-evening make-up

Often, there is very little time to completely redo your make-up before going out in the evening — if the engagement is after work, for instance. So, it saves time to have a good, basic make-up during the day — and to add a few extra touches to give richness and sparkle in the evening. For example, applying a frosted silvery powder eye shadow over your daytime shadow will freshen and enhance your eye make-up. Always re-powder your daytime face with a frosted translucent powder before going out for your evening date. This gives a lively, sparkling effect without being in any way shiny. Re-apply lipstick carefully with a brush, and be more lavish with lipgloss in the evening — artificial light picks up the glossy effect in a most attractive way.

Keep a nail polish deeper than your daytime colour in your handbag. Scratched or chipped nail polish will spoil your evening look — and make you feel untidy too — and it is simple to cover a light polish with just one coat of a darker one when there is no time for a complete manicure.

For evening, use deeper colours to counteract the 'washed out' effects of artificial lights

Remember: artificial lighting is stronger than daylight so a make-up which may have looked fine in sunshine could look washed out and uninteresting at night. Use face-shaders to add evening warmth to your daytime face, and be more lavish with mascara. Build up 'evening eyes' by powdering your lashes between the layers of mascara. Finally, separate the lashes with a dry brush to avoid clogging. (See also Making Up.)

a beautiful smile

Your mouth and teeth

An attractive smile is an important part of beauty. Nothing is more off-putting than dull, bad or discoloured teeth and bad breath, however perfect the rest of a person's face may be.

Dental care at home

Brush teeth thoroughly three times a day after meals. Using a firm tooth-brush, brush your teeth with up and down movements, not with ones that go from side to side. Tackle the back teeth first, both their fronts and backs. Now brush the side teeth, working with up and down strokes. These help to dislodge particles of food by getting the bristles right between the teeth. Finally, brush the front teeth. Rinse your mouth well with an antiseptic mouth-wash several times during the tooth-brushing. Make sure that you massage your gums too with the brush, to stimulate circulation.

If teeth are crooked or full of difficult little crevices, use a round-headed toothbrush to clean them. Use this, too, to push back the gums from the teeth: they may bleed a very little when you do this but that is quite normal. If the bleeding is considerable, however, be sure to consult your dentist without delay. If you have an electric toothbrush, make sure that you replace the brush heads when necessary, every three months or so. And don't think that a 'once over lightly' brushing is all that is necessary. You still have to get into all the crevices. If you use an ordinary tooth brush, don't expect it to last more than six months at the very most.

The whole brushing procedure should take at least three minutes if you do it thoroughly. The choice of toothpaste depends on your preference, of course, but beware of using harsh tooth powders to remove nicotine or other stains as their abrasiveness may damage the enamel on the teeth. It is better to ask your dentist to scale and polish your teeth every six months.

Fresh breath

How do you know whether your breath is fresh? If you've just eaten a highly-seasoned meal or drunk some alcohol, you can be certain that it has made your breath smell. Otherwise, one good way to check is to cup your hand firmly over your mouth and nose, blow out your breath into your hands and breathe in through your nostrils very quickly.

If your breath does not smell fresh for any reason, use a medicated mouthwash and carry an aerosol spray mouth freshener for use during the day. Most important of all — find the cause of the trouble. It could be simply that you are 'out of sorts', it could indicate dental trouble or it could be a sign of stomach disorder. If it persists, consult your dentist.

Diet and your teeth

One of the main causes of the increase in dental troubles in the Western world is diet. Soft, sticky sweets, sugary drinks, cakes and buns all leave sticky deposits on the teeth. These form a breeding-ground for the bacteria that cause dental decay. In children the problem is particularly acute as they tend to eat a lot of sweet foods. And many adults have far too high a proportion of these harmful sweet things in their diet, too. If diet is chosen wisely, it can help to keep teeth white, healthy and beautiful. Here are some easy-to-follow diet ideas:

Always end a meal if possible with fresh, crunchy food such as an apple, a stick of celery or a raw carrot. Eat this after the sweet course. It will ensure that sticky sweet deposits are removed from the vulnerable flat surfaces of the back 'grinding' teeth, where decay can be an all-too-common problem.

Banish sweetened drinks — fruit squashes, fizzy drinks and milk shakes, for example — from your life and replace them with natural, unsweetened fruit juices, milk or water.

Always chew food thoroughly. Remove particles of food from between your teeth with a toothpick after each meal if you are unable to clean your teeth. Bacteria form very quickly indeed.

Beware of too much strong tea or coffee, and of drinks containing iron, like stout. All of them can discolour your teeth.

If you smoke, use a filter-type cigarette holder. Eat an apple every day to counteract nicotine stains.

Replace as many soft, pappy foods as you can with hard, crunchy ones. Have crispbread or crunchy wholewheat bread in place of soft white bread, uncooked vegetables served with a lemon-juice dressing instead of cooked vegetables. Let one meal a day always consist of a crunchy salad.

How your dentist can help

First, get to know him. If you distrust or fear him, find another in whom you have confidence. If you don't do this you may put off dental visits — perhaps subconsciously.

Next, visit the dentist regularly, at least once every six months for a full check-up. If necessary, book an appointment for a thorough scale and polish every few months too. This is particularly necessary if you have the kind of mouth that produces tartar. Tartar is caused by calcium deposits forming between the teeth. It builds up there however often the teeth are cleaned. It can be very harmful, causing gum disorders which are painful and unnecessary. Never try to remove the tartar yourself; let your dentist do it for you.

Most dentists are understanding about the beauty side of mouth care. They will use white fillings in front teeth and sometimes in back teeth, too, to match the natural enamel. Straightening crooked teeth is another aspect of their work. They can also 'crown' unsightly or chipped teeth to give an even, beautiful look. The crowning process can, however, be time-consuming and painful. It consists of filing the tooth to a stump. Most of the hard central core and enamel is then replaced by a synthetic tooth of perfect natural colour and shape. It is a treatment well worth considering, despite the inconvenience, if you have embarrassingly crooked or protruding teeth.

Dentures are very realistic and comfortable now, so that if you do have to have them fitted, it is not a drastic matter. They do, however, need regular after-care and meticulous cleaning for hygiene and beauty.

A beautiful smile is a marvellous beauty asset. Care for your teeth by brushing regularly—and see your dentist often

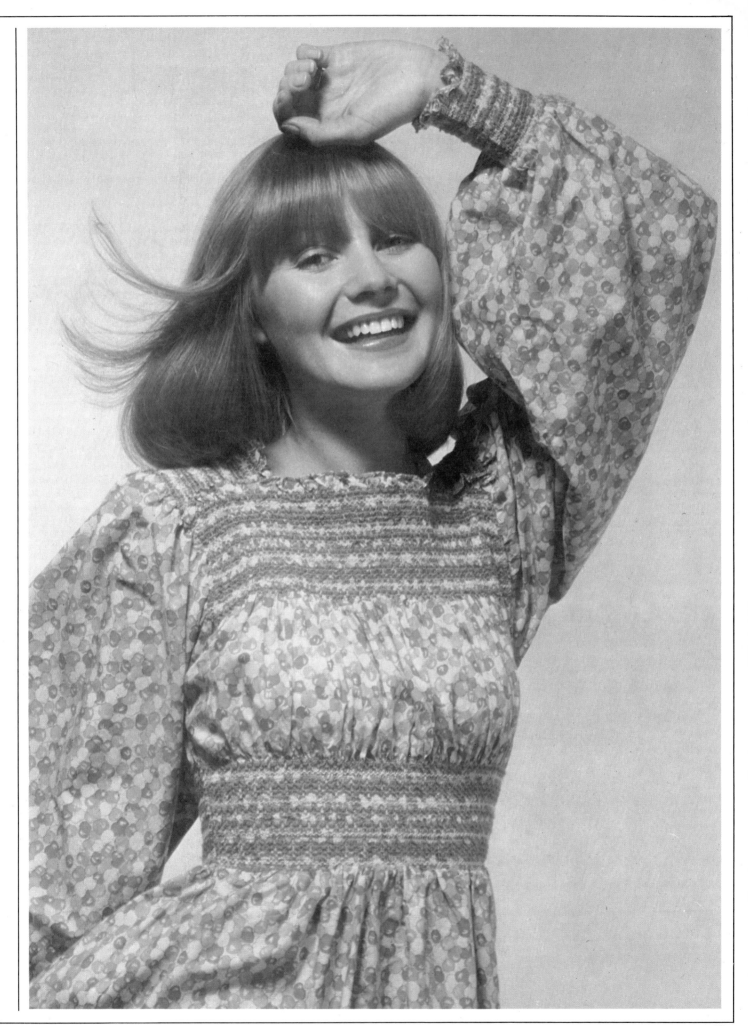

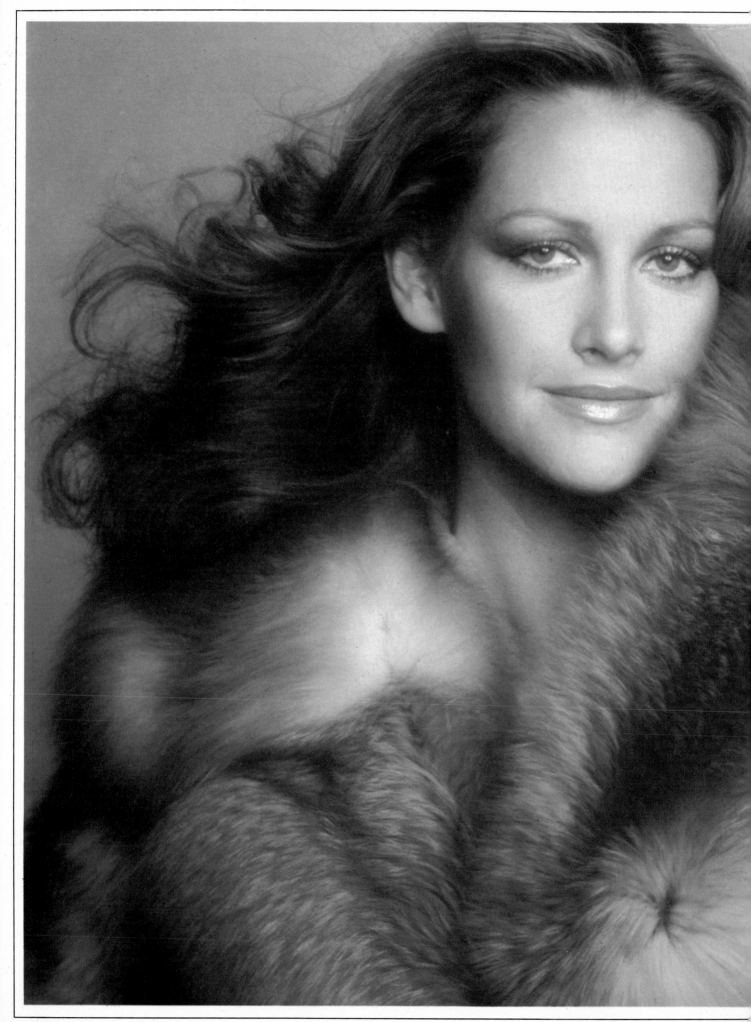

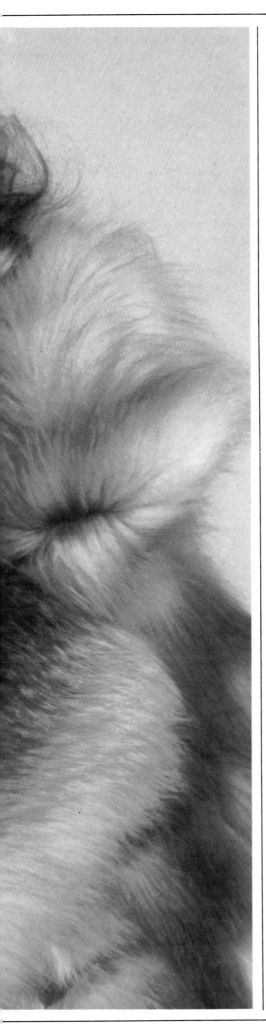

hair - bright & shiny

Lovely, shining hair is one of a woman's greatest beauty assets. So it makes sense to know something about the way hair grows, what it is made of and the conditions it needs to stay healthy. Hair tends to be the body's 'barometer', indicating good health or the lack of it. The barometer may swing up and down fairly rapidly, and that can be annoying. However, with care you can control the health and temperament of your hair to a great extent. But first you need to know a good deal about it:

What hair is made of

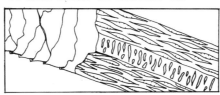

If you cut through a single hair, then magnified the cut end under a very powerful microscope, you will see that there is a distinct central core or medulla, surrounded by another layer called the cortex and then the cuticle which looks like overlapping roof tiles. The hair is made of a protein-based substance called keratin. Variations of the same substance form toe and finger nails.

How hair grows

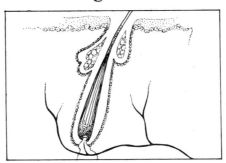

The hair shaft grows from a snug cavity called the hair follicle. If you were to pluck a hair from your head and look at the root end under the microscope, you would see that the end is rather more bulbous-looking, and that it is covered with blood. The hair is fed by blood flowing to the follicle — which is why good circulation in the scalp is vital to healthy hair. Hair grows at the rate of about $\frac{1}{2}$ inch a month, or six inches a year, although the rate slows down a little with age. This means that the ends of long hair are really quite elderly: a girl with hair measuring 18 inches or so has three-year-old hair ends. No wonder the ends of dry hair so often become brittle and split. They may have been through quite a lot in their lifetime.

What makes hair shine

A group of sebaceous glands is situated about halfway up the hair follicle. These secrete sebum, the natural hair lubricant which makes hair lively and shiny. As the hair shaft grows, it is coated with sebum, which should flow freely the full length of the shaft. It can be prevented from flowing down the hair shaft by dandruff encrustations on the surface of the scalp, or because the sebaceous glands are not producing enough of it. In either event, a dry hair condition occurs. Obviously, the sebum must flow a considerable way to get to the ends of long hair — which is why they are very often dry. When the sebaceous glands are over-active, a greasy hair condition occurs. This over-activity can be due to bad diet or glandular activity in the body, rather as over-active glands can cause acne in teenagers.

Why hair falls out

The lifespan of a hair can be anything from several months to several years, depending on how it is treated and how healthy the scalp and hair condition are. On a healthy head, new hairs are growing from the hair follicles all the time. So, although a hundred or so hairs may come out in a single day, your hair won't become thinner. The trouble starts when new hair does *not* form in the follicle, perhaps because there is inadequate blood supply, or because glandular or hormonal activity in the body is preventing healthy growth. Experts in hair — trichologists — believe that this hormonal activity is greatest amongst worried or over-ambitious middle-aged men. Stimulating scalp circulation and accelerating sluggish blood-flow to the follicles can help, but there are no miraculous cures for baldness (alopaecia). In fact, the condition is now becoming commoner than it once was among women, as they grow more career-minded.

Hair pigment and curl

The colour of your hair is determined by hereditary factors. If your parents were both fair, then you are likely to be fair too; if one was dark and one was fair, then you could be one or the other or a mixture of both.

The genes which decide your natural hair pigment are also responsible for deciding whether your hair will be curly or straight. Curly hair is actually 'curled' beneath the surface of the scalp: the shape of the hair follicle itself forces the growing hair into kinks and waves.

Nature, however, often seems to have a good eye for colour and form, providing the hair colour which harmonizes with skin tone, the softness of waves to set off a strong face. In the majority of cases, the natural hair colouring is the most pleasing to the eye, although it sometimes needs a little artificial addition to give it depth. Radical changes to hair colour and degree of curliness very rarely suit the person who makes them.

Caring for your hair

Hair is a precious beauty asset so it deserves good care. First, decide what is your type of hair.

Hair type

Normal hair is shiny yet not greasy, and fairly easy to manage. Although it may fly about a little the day after a set, it soon settles down and will stay looking good for about a week before it becomes slightly sticky to the touch and dirty-looking.

Greasy hair looks good for a day or two after shampooing, but then quickly becomes lank. Groups of hairs cling together in unattractive strands and the scalp feels dirty.

Dry hair is difficult to control after shampooing, looks dull and has ends that are dry and split. Even just before shampooing, the ends look dry. The scalp too feels dry and sometimes itchy.

Greasy dry hair is usually fairly long and the hair nearest the scalp is greasy while the ends are dry. Just after shampooing, the hair looks good, except for the ends. These seem difficult to set smoothly and look split and lighter in colour than the roots. By the time that the scalp feels dirty enough for another shampoo (after only a few days), the ends probably look quite good.

It is very irritating.

Here is how to care for all four hair types:

Normal hair Wash one a week with a mild shampoo. Many of the shampoos on the market contain harsh detergents to produce the frothy lather which people seem to feel makes their hair cleaner. It doesn't — but it can often strip the natural sebum from the hair and spoil its condition. So search for a very mild baby or herbal shampoo which suits your hair. Apply a little to the scalp, rub in well with the tips of your fingers, then allow the shampoo to run down the hair shafts. Do not rub the ends of the hair vigorously. Rinse, re-apply and work up a little lather. Rinse thoroughly. If the hair occasionally looks as though it needs a conditioner, mix two egg-yolks with a cup of luke warm water and beat together. Massage into the scalp, then cover your hair with a plastic bag and leave it in place for 10 minutes. After that, rinse hair thoroughly with lukewarm water, then shampoo it.

Greasy hair Wash it often, preferably just before it starts looking and feeling sticky. This may mean three times a week or more. Frequent washing will not make greasy hair worse. On the other hand, if it stays greasy, the grease can cause spots to appear on your face and back.

Choose a lemon-based shampoo and pay particular attention to the scalp when massaging the shampoo in. Rinse very thoroughly, and add a little vinegar to the final rinsing water to leave the hair squeaking clean.

Pay very careful attention to your diet. Avoid fatty and fried foods, salad oils, sticky buns and sweets. Increase your intake of protein-rich foods like eggs, meat, fish or cheese, salad vegetables, and of citrus fruits and unsweetened fruit juices. Drink plenty of water, too. Occasionally, excessively greasy hair may be connected with poor thyroid-gland function and stress. Try to relax more, to 'switch off' by taking outdoor exercise.

If you have greasy hair, it makes sense to choose a hair style which can be set quickly at home. Simpler still is a good cut which can be brushed into shape quickly after each shampoo. Don't choose a complicated style if you know that you're going to have to wash your hair several times a week — and invest in a good hair-dryer to save time, too. It's more important to have clean, shiny hair than curls and waves. Long hair can look lovely, but only if it's clean. Never, leave long hair greasy and lank.

A dry shampoo If a sudden invitation finds you with dull, droopy hair and no time to shampoo it, try a dry shampoo. Divide your hair into sections and fluff a little fuller's earth through each section. Rub in well and leave for 10 minutes. Brush out thoroughly with a clean brush. You will find that the fuller's earth has absorbed most of the grease and dirt, leaving your hair soft and shining. Dab a little cologne on the scalp to give it fragrance.

Dry hair Wash once a week with a cream shampoo, and apply a conditioner afterwards. Remember to rinse the conditioner off very thoroughly to avoid stickiness.

Every two weeks, try the following treatment: warm a cupful of olive oil, and saturate the hair. Cover your hair with a plastic bag secured with hair-grips [bobby pins]. Cover the bag with a warmed towel, wrapped turban-fashion. Leave the olive-oil conditioner on for half an hour, then rinse away thoroughly and shampoo your hair in the normal way.

If your hair tends to be fly-away, avoid using harsh lacquers [hair spray], even though it is tempting to do so. Instead put a dab of cream conditioner on your brush before styling your hair. Lacquer [hair spray] will only tend to aggravate the dryness.

If your scalp is dry too, stimulate the flow of sebum and blood to the hair follicles with a do-it-yourself scalp massage. Cup your hands with fingers a little apart and press the pads of your fingers hard down on your scalp. Massage firmly but gently, moving the scalp itself, not your fingers. Now move your hands to another part of your scalp, and repeat the process. Make sure that your diet is high in protein — fish, meat, eggs and cheese — and that it includes vegetable oils. A good way to treat your hair from the inside is to use an olive-oil dressing on salads.

Greasy dry hair Wash as soon as the scalp feels itchy, but use a very mild shampoo and do not rub the shampoo into the dry ends. Instead, concentrate on massaging the shampoo into the scalp, then let a little run down the hair shafts. Rinse. (The ends of your hair will become even more dry if you over-wash them.)

Afterwards, use a conditioner on the ends only, and rinse it off thoroughly. Have the dry ends trimmed regularly. Keep your scalp scrupulously clean between shampoos by making partings all over your head and rubbing each one with a piece of cologne-soaked cotton wool [cotton].

diet for healthy hair

The beauty of hair—like the beauty of the whole body—depends on good health. Since hair is made from a form of protein, a high protein diet can help to make it grow strong and healthy. People who lose hair temporarily in accidents are usually given a high protein diet of meat, fish, eggs, cheese and milk by doctors to ensure that the new hair grows thick and strong.

The valuable vitamins of the 'B' complex are also important for hair health, and one of the best sources of Vitamin B is brewer's yeast. Trichologists often treat dull and falling hair with a course of brewer's yeast tablets, up to as many as 6 a day. Another good source of Vitamin B is liver, so make sure your diet includes at least one liver meal a week.

Minerals important for the health of your hair include iron, copper and iodine. Although iron and copper are present in everyday foods like meat and leafy green vegetables, iodine is often very low in the average diet. Seafood is the best source, so step up your intake of fish and shellfish.

If you have greasy hair, banish fried, greasy and fatty foods from your diet and concentrate on green vegetables and salads, meat, fresh fish, liver, eggs and cheese. For dry hair, add a little vegetable oil (on salads) to the same basic diet, but avoid fried food, since it may cause skin troubles.

Dandruff can be a problem for dry, normal or greasy hair. A well-balanced diet and good general health are essential for getting rid of dandruff permanently. Anti-dandruff shampoo may clear the scalp of the encrustations of dandruff for a time, but they recur.

Breakfast, every day
1 egg, boiled or poached
1 slice wholewheat bread
Tea or coffee
1 brewer's yeast tablet

Monday
Mid-morning
Glass of mixed vegetable juice with a little wheat germ stirred into it
Lunch
Mixed salad vegetables*
Cheese or cold meat
1 orange
Tea or coffee
1 brewer's yeast tablet
Evening meal
Grilled [broiled] cod
Carrots
Green beans
Apple pie made with wholewheat flour
A little cream
Tea or coffee
1 brewer's yeast tablet

Tuesday
Mid-morning
Large glass of orange juice with a little wheat germ stirred into it
Lunch
2-egg omelette
Salad of watercress, grated cabbage, grated carrot*
Slice of wholewheat bread with a little butter
1 apple
Tea or coffee
1 brewer's yeast tablet
Evening meal
Grilled [broiled] liver and bacon
Grilled [broiled] tomatoes
Brussel sprouts
Natural yogurt with a few raisins added to it
Tea or coffee
1 brewer's yeast tablet

Wednesday
Mid-morning
Large glass of tomato juice with a little wheat germ stirred into it
Lunch
Grilled [broiled] pork chop
Salad of lettuce, cucumber, tomato, watercress*
Fresh orange and grapefruit segments with a spoonful of honey
Tea or coffee
1 brewer's yeast tablet
Evening meal
Steak and kidney pie made with wholewheat pastry crust

Cauliflower
Grilled [broiled] tomato
Small piece of hard cheese
Tea or coffee
1 brewer's yeast tablet

Thursday
Mid-morning
Large glass of milk with 1 tablespoon honey added to it
Lunch
Small grilled [broiled] hamburger steak
Watercress*
Grilled [broiled] tomato
Natural yogurt with chopped apple and raisins added to it
Tea or coffee
1 brewer's yeast tablet
Evening meal
Grilled [broiled] lamb chop with dill
Brown rice
Broccoli
Fruit salad
Tea or coffee
1 brewer's yeast tablet

Friday
Mid-morning
Large glass of mixed vegetable juice with a little wheat germ stirred into it
Lunch
Grilled [broiled] fish
Salad of watercress, lettuce, cucumber, chopped chives*
Baked apple
Tea or coffee
1 brewer's yeast tablet
Evening meal
Cauliflower cheese
Grilled [broiled] tomatoes
2 small boiled potatoes
Egg custard
Tea or coffee
1 brewer's yeast tablet

Weekend
Eat normally, remembering to take the 3 brewer's yeast tablets daily. Avoid all fried and fatty foods, sticky sweets and alcohol.
*Have an olive oil dressing for dry hair; lemon juice for greasy hair.

choosing a hair style

The right hair style can make any woman look more attractive — it takes the eye away from any physical flaws, and draws it to something pleasing. The choice of a hair style depends on a number of basic principles:

Know Your Face Shape

First, take all your hair back severely from your face. Now, study the contours carefully in a mirror. Is your face round, square, heart-shaped, long, heavy-jawed? A long, honest look will soon tell you, but if necessary, ask a friend for a candid assessment to confirm your own judgement. Now, use that basic knowledge of your face shape when you choose a hairstyle — regardless of the whims of fashion! You will almost certainly find, anyway, that there is a variation of a fashionable style that is right for you.

First and Foremost—The Right Cut

Go to the best hairdresser you can afford for your new hair style. If possible, take with you a magazine picture showing the kind of style you think you would like. Decide firmly before you go how short you want your hair. Take advice from the hairdresser, of course, but do not be bullied into having your hair cut too short. A skilful hairdresser can make thin hair look thicker with the right cut. He can also advise you on perming and colouring techniques. Ask him to show you how he sets your new style so that you can copy the method at home.

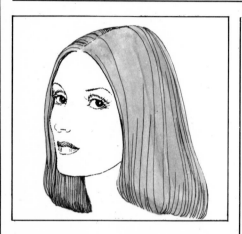

Round face To lengthen and slim the contours of your face, choose a straightish style with a centre parting, with no fringes [bangs], curls or waves to break the line. The ends of your hair should be below chin level, and cut evenly, not in a ragged line. Avoid any height above the browline or width at ear level.

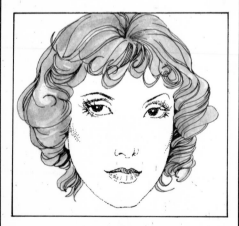

Long face A fringe [bangs] or soft half-fringe will help to shorten your face, and a little width at the sides will broaden it successfully. Keep your hair fairly short — long hair with a long face tends to 'pull down' your whole appearance.

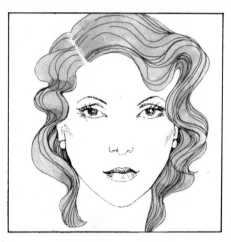

Heart-shaped face With a fairly broad forehead and a pointed chin, you need softness at the temples and fullness just below ear level. This is one one of the easier face-shapes for hair styling but avoid a centre parting, which will tend to emphasize your pointed chin.

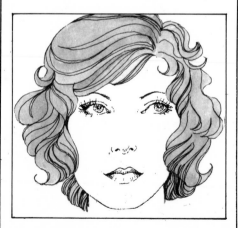

Square face Soften the brow and jawline with a curvy style. Have fronds or a fall of hair at the temples, and hair curling forward on to the jawbone. You can take an asymetrical style with a side parting. Avoid styles where the hair is severely drawn back from the face. If your hair is limp, you may need a light perm [permanent] to hold the movement which is most flattering you to face shape.

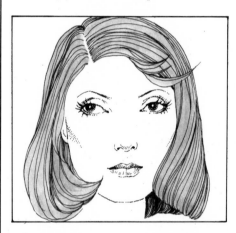

Heavy jawline Make sure your hair falls forward at jaw level to hide the heavy line. Balance the width of your jaw with height and width at the top of your head, too, otherwise your face will have an exaggeratedly triangular look.

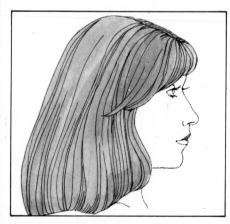

Prominent nose Keep the hairline at the temples soft, with a short fringe or half-fringe [bangs], and make sure that there is fullness at the back of your head to balance your profile. Avoid chignons or very short, severe styles.

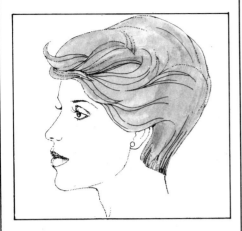

Short neck Balance a short neck by wearing your hair short with height on the crown. Never wear your hair below chin level, or your neck will tend to disappear altogether!

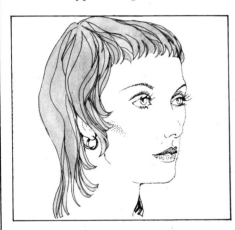

Low forehead Choose a style which brushes the hair back from the brow and have a short fringe [bangs], taken from a high parting on the crown of the head.

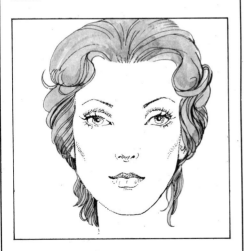

Big ears Cover your ears with soft waves or a smooth, full fall of hair. If you prefer to wear your hair short, make sure that the strands in front of your ears are left long enough to brush back and cover them and

that the sides are left full and thick by the hairdresser.

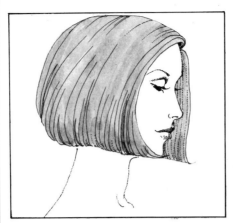

Receding chin Have your hair cut to jaw level and swinging forward to cover your chin when it is seen in profile.

Know your figure type

Your figure matters almost as much as the shape of your face when you are choosing a hair style. Look at yourself in a full-length mirror, slowly and carefully from all angles.

Tall and slim You're lucky — most hairstyles will suit you. However, avoid really short hair which could give you a 'pinhead' look.

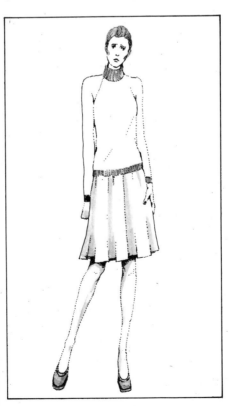

Tall and plump Balance your shape with medium-length hair, cut to give a little width. Long hair will make you look clumsy, very short hair will

be unflattering — and make you appear even plumper.

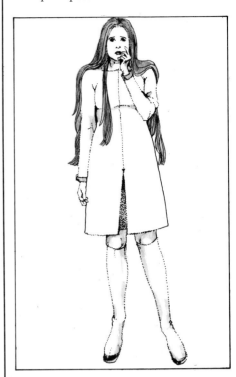

Short and slim You can wear most styles — but avoid very long hair or very full styles, which could make you look top-heavy.

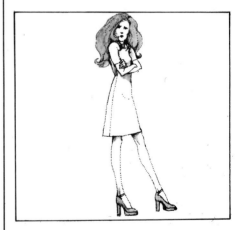

Short and plump Hair cut to jaw level is best for you. Keep it fairly smooth to avoid having a 'dimpled dolly' look.

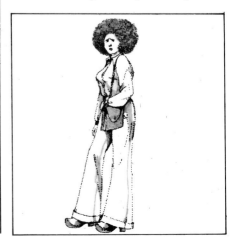

care for your hair

You will need: towel, setting lotion for fine, fly-away hair, hair pins, hair net, hair dryer, soft brush, tail comb, rollers in different sizes (open mesh rollers, without spikes or brushes inside them, are best for quick drying without tangles).

Washing First shampoo your hair, then wrap it in a towel and allow this to soak up the excess moisture. That is better for the hair than vigorous drying with a towel since hair is very vulnerable when wet. It tends to snap more easily, ends split more quickly and the hair becomes very stretchy. So, handle it with care.

After about ten minutes, remove the towel and comb the hair through very gently. Start with the ends, combing downwards, then working backwards towards the scalp. If hair is combed from the scalp downwards, tangles will build up on the way down and reach the tugging stage very quickly.

If you have very long or thick hair, partly dry it before setting. Hold the hair dryer well away from the hair, gently ruffling it with your fingers to allow the hot air to penetrate. Comb through very gently once more, using setting lotion if you like.

Setting Divide hair into sections and set one section at a time, securing the other sections with clips so that they do not get in your way. Take each strand of hair in your left hand and hold it at right angles to the scalp as you put in the roller with your right hand. This is to ensure maximum 'bounce' from your set. Be careful to tuck the ends of the hair in smoothly (the tail comb is useful for this) before you roll up firmly but not too tightly. You may find that the small fronds of hair at the hairline or the nape of the neck are easier to set with clips or a strip of sticky tape. Aim for a very neat set. Cover with a hair net.

Drying Now dry carefully, holding

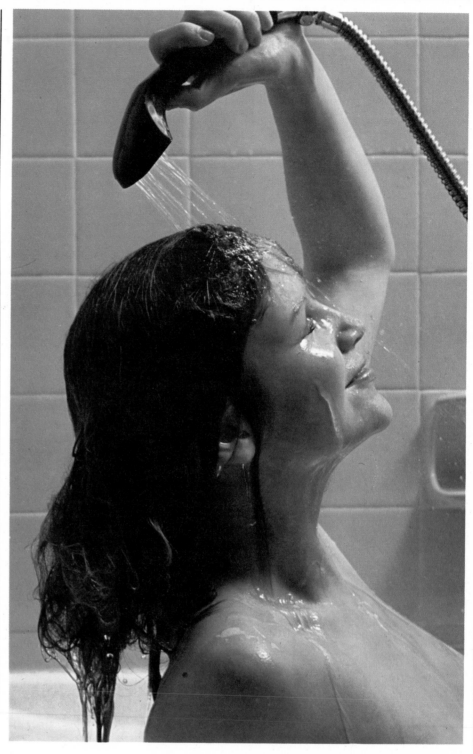

the dryer at least one foot away from the hair. You may find that a hood-type dryer is easier to use, leaving your hands free for reading, knitting or needlework.

To test whether your hair is thoroughly dry, undo one of the front rollers. Allow the hair to cool before removing all the other rollers slowly and carefully. Do not tug.

Brush the hair into shape gently. Its natural bounce should enough body without back-combing [teasing], which is very bad for your hair. Hard-to-hold hair will benefit from a beer setting lotion: simply dip your comb

Regular shampooing is a necessary part of beauty care, and clean shining hair is a great morale booster.

in a little stale beer and comb it through each section before you roll it up.

Rollers Smooth plastic rollers are the best choice. Metal rollers become very hot under the hot air from a dryer, and may damage the hair ends which are rolled right next to them. Rollers with bristles inside or little points or knobs on the outside often become tangled in the hair and are difficult, then, to remove without breaking the hair.

how to roll it up & comb it out

Follow the roller sketches shown here to set the hairstyles pictured in the Hair Colouring section

1. *Use clips for the pincurls which form the soft fringe [bangs] of this style, medium-sized rollers on top and sides, smaller rollers at the nape of the neck. Ask your hairdresser for a layered cut for this style — about 6 inches at the top, 10 inches at the bottom*

2. *The large forward-swinging curls at the sides of this style are set with sticky tape. The top hair is brushed smoothly back from the brow and fastened with an invisible hair pin, colour-matched to the hair. Ask your hairdresser for a blunt-cut bob, shaped slightly into the nape of the neck*

3. *Set longer or medium-length hair on large rollers all over (hair turned under) and brush out smoothly with a centre parting. If hair is long, twist it into the loose coils shown and fasten with hair pins. If it is shorter, grip neatly in place and use softly-coiled hairpieces instead, fastened securely to the base*

4. *Make a centre parting and set as shown in the sketches. Brush out smoothly and let side curls fall naturally forward. If your hair is long, twist the back hair into a smooth coil and fasten in place with hair pins. If it is short, 'gather' the back hair together with hair pins and add a false 'bun' or coiled hairpiece*

5. *Make a centre parting at the front of your hair and comb the rest back. Set as shown in the diagram, using one big roller for the top hair and tiny rollers for the hair at the nape of the neck. For the characteristic pageboy look, ask your hairdresser to cut the hair at the back about 2 inches longer than the sides. This style suits medium-long or very long hair*

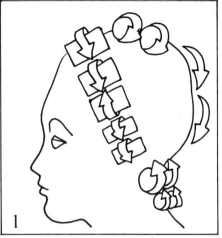

1

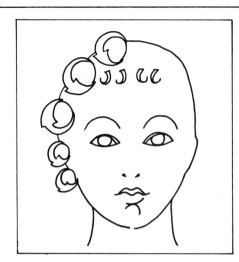

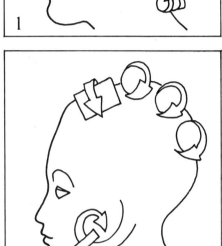

2

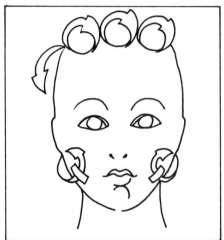

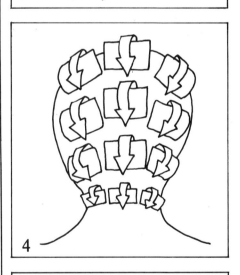

4

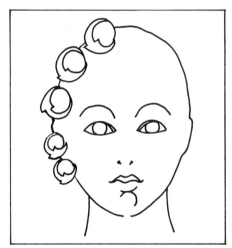

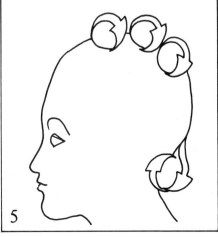

5

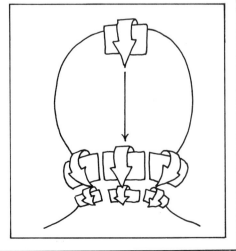

hair colouring

The cells which contain the colour pigments of the hair are in the cortex, just below the cuticle, or surface, of the hair. It is in the cortex that hair colouring changes take place when chemical colourants and bleaches are applied.

Colour with caution

If you feel that nature can be improved upon, or you want a change, then consider trying a hair colourant. It can give a great lift to your whole appearance, and hair colouring techniques now are far gentler and more sophisticated than they were a few years ago. But do not make the mistake of trying a really radical colour change — dark brown to blond, for example. A drastic change is unlikely to suit your skin tone, and the cost of keeping up the colour change would be tremendous. In addition, to bleach hair from dark brown to blonde involves stripping the pigment from the cortex with a strong bleaching agent, then toning with a colourant. The process is harsh and with the best will in the world, your hairdresser will be unable to avoid overlapping the bleach when colouring the regrowth of hair. The twice bleached hair will be brittle and will probably split or break.

Here are useful points to keep in mind:

1 Hair darker than your natural colour may be aging. Lighter, brighter tones are usually more flattering than really heavy, dark shades. Try a wig in the colour of your choice before making up your mind.

2 A new hair colour will mean a completely new make-up, and possibly even a new wardrobe too. The lipstick that suited you as a blonde is unlikely to look good when you become a redhead. Take a range of lipsticks and eye shadows to the hairdresser who colours your hair, and re-do your make-up before you leave. If you don't, you may hate the new hair colour before you've given yourself a chance to get used to it. Another point: if you have a wardrobe full of brightly coloured clothes which gave you added colour when your hair was a light brown, you may find that they look too overpowering when you become a streaked blonde.

So, be prepared for some extra expense.

3 Hair colour needs careful upkeep. Regrowth looks messy and unflattering. Consider just how much time you will have to spend at the hairdresser each week before you take the plunge.

4 Hair colourants can have disastrous effects on out-of-condition hair. If your hair is dry, brittle or lank or if you have just got over an illness or had a baby, postpone having a new colour until your hair is in tiptop shape once more. Your hairdresser will not and cannot take the responsibility if the colour goes wrong because your hair starts as bad raw material.

5 Hair which has just had a perm [permanent] may not take colour, and newly-coloured hair may not perm well, either. Keep appointments for perm [permanent] and hair-colouring well apart. Three to four weeks is a good interval.

Types of hair colourant

Rinses and brighteners These give a 'lift' to the natural hair shade but they wash out with the next shampoo. They are easy to apply at home. A red rinse on dull brown hair will bring out pretty lights, and a honey-gold rinse on blond hair looks lovely, too. But no point in using a light rinse on dark hair — it just won't 'take'.

Semi-permanent colourants These are designed to last through 6-8 shampoos. Choose the colour carefully if you are doing the job yourself. Make sure that you put a large old towel around your shoulders while the hair is wet, as these colourants do stain. They work by coating the hair shaft with colour and do not contain a bleach. If you have thin or lank hair, the use of a semi-permanent colourant will add body and bounce.

Permanent colourants These contain a bleaching agent which strips the existing pigment from the hair shaft. This leaves the hair porous, brittle and spongy — ready to absorb the new colour. This will last as long as the hair itself, although the actual pigment may fade and need retouching. Hair which is coloured with a permanent colourant needs special care in strong sunlight since the sun may continue the bleaching action started by the bleaching agent. As a result the hair may become lighter, brittle and dry-looking. Always cover coloured hair in strong sunshine and avoid contact with salt water. Do not use a colourant which hurts the scalp or produces dandruff-like encrustations on it.

Streaking Try streaking your hair at home only if your hair is already quite fair or a light brown colour. Several firms now make a do-it-yourself kit for streaking, consisting of a bleaching preparation, plastic cap and toner. Brush your hair well. Put on the plastic cap and bring through the small holes in it fine strands of hair (about six hairs to each strand). Apply the bleach to these strands only. The rest of your hair is protected by the cap. Leave the bleach to work according to the maker's instructions. Rinse off the bleach. Remove the cap and shampoo your hair in the usual way. After shampooing, apply toner. Leave it to work according to the maker's instructions. Rinse thoroughly.

Natural colourants Before chemists concocted the sophisticated hair dyes which are now available, women coloured their hair with natural plants and roots. Some are still used today, but they do require considerable skill and care in use:

When experimenting with home hair dyes, always try out the effect on a cutting of end hair first. The ends of your hair are the most porous part and accept the dye more readily — so you can see the full effect before you take the plunge.

Henna dyes dark hair a reddish colour. However, the exact colour result is very difficult to predict so a test dye is absolutely essential. The dye actually coats the hair shaft, giving bounce and body to the hair. It cannot be used on hair which is already coloured, or on fair hair, for it can turn this very carroty indeed! The usual recipe for the dye is: 2 cups henna powder, 1 cup warm water, 1 teaspoon pure vinegar. Stir to a thick paste, let this stand for 1 hour, then put it into the top of a double boiler and stir until the water in the bottom of the saucepan bubbles freely. Let the mixture stand for another hour, then massage it into your hair, wearing rubber gloves to protect your hands. Leave the henna on your head for 3-6 hours, depending on the depth of colour required. Wash off and rinse very, very thoroughly. Usually, a conditioner is required after henna dyeing.

Saffron will also give hair a reddish tint. Make an infusion of saffron in warm water and use as a rinse after shampooing.

Camomile will lighten mousy hair. Infuse a handful of flowers in a cup of boiling water, leave for a few hours, then strain. Use as a rinse after shampooing.

(Both saffron and camomile flowers are available from health stores.)

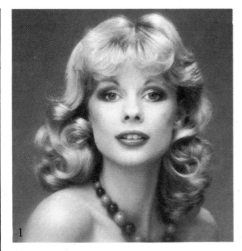

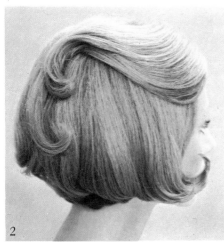

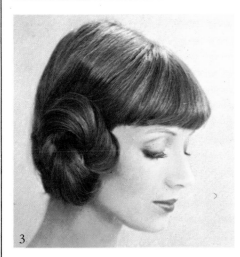

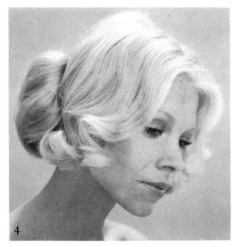

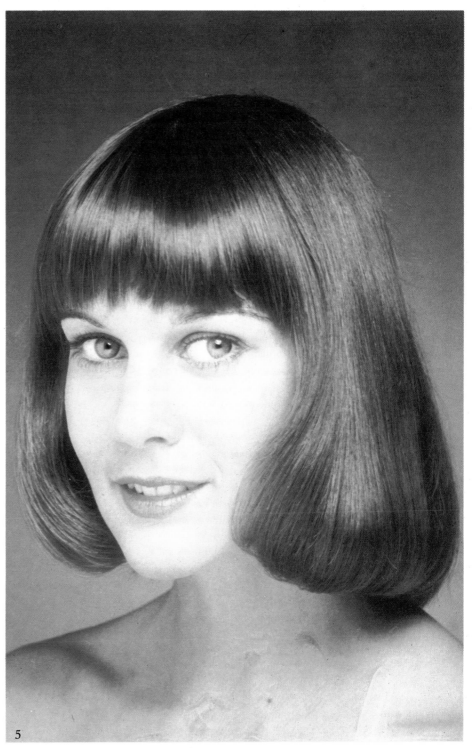

Use your natural hair colour as a guide when choosing a semi-permanent or permanent hair tint. Drastic changes are unlikely to be successful, since your skin-tone and the colour of your eyes will probably look strange with the new shade. Remember too that lightening your hair is less aging than going darker

1. *Fair or 'mousey' hair takes well to permanent lightening. Use a mild bleaching preparation plus a toner, or an all-in-one bleaching and toning product. Streaking is also pretty on fair hair—and it adds body*

2. *Light brown hair can be lightened just a few shades and tinted to a warm, pretty honey colour*

3. *Medium or dark brown hair becomes glossy and more manageable with a semi-permanent tint. Play up red highlights if you like*

4. *Very light brown or blonde hair can be lightened still more for a pale, Scandanavian look. Use conditioner often, though*

5. *Add depth to medium or light brown hair with a darker brown tint. Or, lighten dark hair to a warm medium shade*

care for your skin

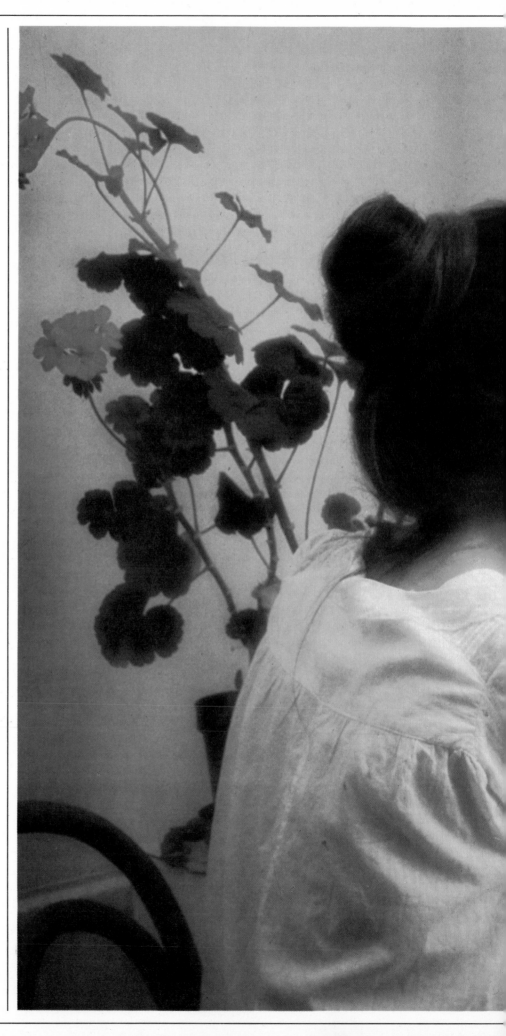

Make-up applied to an imperfect skin will improve its appearance. Make-up applied to a good, well-cared-for skin will make it beautiful. The basis of lasting good looks is regular, thorough skin care.

Before planning your skin care routine, it is good to know something about the construction of the skin itself.

The structure of the skin

Most people think of the skin's surface as one single layer. In fact there are three main layers: the epidermis, the cutis (or corum) and the sub-cutis. The epidermis — the top layer — is itself divided into five cell layers: the horny layer (the topmost layer), the glossy layer, the granular cell layer, the prickle cell layer and the basal cell layer (see the diagram.)

EPIDERMIS	Horny Layer	
	Glossy Layer	Keratin Membrane
		Granular Cell Layer
		Prickle Cell Layer
		Basal Cell Layer
	CUTIS OR CORIUM	
	SUB-CUTIS	

The lower cell layers have a low water content and the upper cell layers have a high water content. They are separated by a membrane called the keratin membrane situated between the glossy cell layer and the granular cell layer. Together, the prickle cell layer and the basal cell layer form the germ layer.

The topmost layer of the skin (the horny layer) is constantly renewed from the germ layer. New cells are formed

Regular, deep-cleansing is vital for a soft, unblemished skin. Use two applications of cleanser for a thorough job

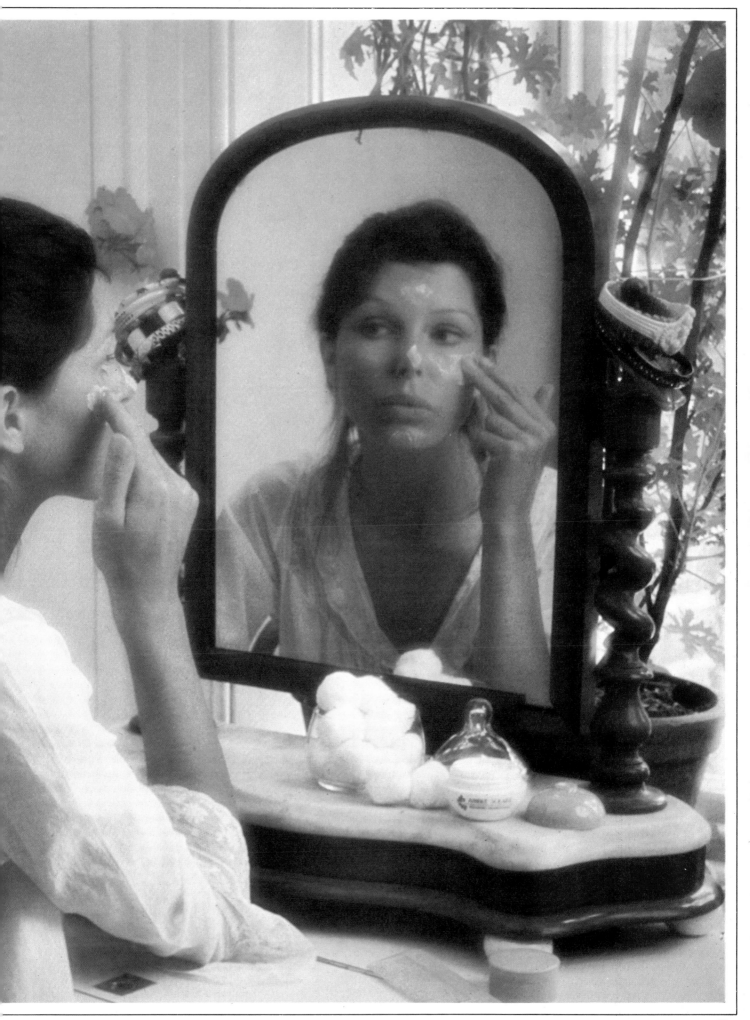

and rise to the horny layer over a period of about three weeks. When they reach the top and are exposed to the air, a chemical change takes place. They are converted into keratin particles, highly resistant to water, overlapping rather like roof tiles. The particles are held together by a waxy, water-binding substance.

The horny layer consists of 10 percent water and this moisture is vital to the preservation of the softness and suppleness of the skin and of its elasticity. If the moisture content is lost (in a process known as dehydration), the top layer becomes brittle, dull and lifeless and lines appear in it. Exposure to intense heat or cold or the use of very drying make-up or soaps can all help to dehydrate the skin. This is why moisturizing is so important.

In the cutis (or corum) are situated the sebaceous and sweat glands. The sebaceous glands secrete sebum which helps to form the grease and acid protection on the horny surface of the skin. The sebaceous glands can occasionally become over-active. This is due either to the presence of a male hormone called androgen or to emotional disturbance. From the over-activity the condition called acne can arise.

As the skin ages, the moisturizing action slows down and the blood circulation becomes less efficient. The skin loses much of its elasticity and resilience and its lines become fixed. Regular, careful moisturizing (especially between the ages of 25 and 40) can help to delay this process.

Diet and your skin

Skin must be constantly renewed to be healthy. This means that cell movement must be encouraged by good circulation. Vitamin C, helping to purify and vitalize the blood stream, is vital for good skin. It is to be found in fruits (especially the citrus fruits like oranges, tangerines, lemons, grapefruit), green vegetables and potatoes. For healthy formation skin also needs Vitamin B2 from fresh vegetables, milk and wholemeal [wholewheat] bread.

It was thought that chocolate and sweets were responsible for spotty [blemished] skin, but this theory has been discarded by skin specialists. However, they now suggest that people who indulge in sweet snacks are unlikely to eat sufficient fruit to provide the Vitamin C which the skin needs so much. The important point here is that Vitamin C cannot be stored by the body and so it must be supplied daily. There is evidence, however, that fried and greasy foods and alcohol can cause blemishes and blotchiness on the skin's surface. So, it is wise to keep these to a minimum in your diet. Alcohol and coffee or tea all interfere with the body's ability to assimilate Vitamin B. If you replace them by unsweetened orange or grapefruit juice whenever possible, you are doing your skin—and your whole body—a service.

What is your skin type?

It is an over-simplification to divide all skins into four groups, since every skin is highly individual with its own individual characteristics. However, for the purposes of choosing your skin care routine and buying the right skin care products, your skin will fall into one of these categories:

Normal skin A smooth, good tempered skin with no enlarged pores or flaky dead cells. There may be the occasional pimple (just before menstruation when increased hormonal activity causes the sebaceous glands to be over-active), but acne is certainly not a problem. Normal skin will line in time, but regular moisturizing will help to slow down the process.

Dry skin This skin is flaky and dull-looking, especially on the cheeks and around the eyes. Even in the teens fine lines may appear here and at the corners of the mouth on a very dry skin. Dry skin becomes reddened and sore in cold weather, too. However, spots [blemishes] very rarely appear.

Oily skin If you hold a tissue on an un-made-up oily skin, then remove it, you will notice that the tissue is slightly greasy. Oily skin is shiny, with a coarse texture and open pores on the chin and round the sides of the nose. Spots [blemishes] or even acne may appear on the chin, cheekbones and forehead. Make-up turns shiny-looking after only a few hours.

Combination skin This is a very common skin-type. There are coarse, open pores round the nose and on the chin, but the skin on the cheekbones is dry and flaky. The forehead is often greasy too, and so the greasy area of the face forms a central panel from the forehead, over the nose and down the chin. The eye area is dryish, and fine lines may appear there quite early in life. Pimples will always appear on the greasy areas — the chin, the sides of the nose or the forehead.

This can be a troublesome type of skin since it seems to combine the worst features of both dry and oily skins. It needs to be tackled with two totally different skin-care routines.

How to care for your skin

Cleansing, toning and nourishing are the three basic requirements of a good skin-care programme. Even the oiliest skin needs nourishing and protecting as well as very thorough, deep cleansing. If skin care is neglected, the epidermis will suffer. Lack of regular cleansing, for instance, will cause a build-up of dead cells and stale make-up on its horny top layer.

Each skin type needs a different kind of care.

Normal skin *Cleanse* with a light cleansing cream applied in generous blobs on cheeks, chin, forehead and throat. Always tuck your hair into a bandeau before putting on the cream to avoid making your hair greasy. Massage the cream into your face with light upwards strokes, then remove with cotton wool [cotton]. Repeat the whole procedure. Avoid the eye area as you work. Now apply eye make-up remover cream to closed eyes, using a very small amount. Wipe away gently with cotton wool [cotton]; most tissues are too harsh for this delicate area.

This cleansing routine must be followed every night. In the morning, use a gentle, unperfumed soap and water or, if you prefer, cleanse with your skin cream again. A normal skin will not be adversely affected by water, but do make sure that all traces of soap are rinsed away thoroughly and that skin is moisturized afterwards.

Tone with a light skin tonic to refresh the skin and close pores after cleansing. Never choose a harsh astringent lotion for this purpose: a rosewater-based product is best. Dab a little toning lotion on cotton wool [cotton] lightly over your face without dragging the skin.

Moisturize with a light, liquid moisturizer applied sparingly: heavy creams are unnecessary for your skin. Put this on with the very tips of your fingers. Always apply after cleansing and toning at night and before putting on make-up in the morning. The moisturizer forms an invisible, protective barrier which helps to keep make-up fresh for longer, and also stops the keratin particles of the horny top layer of the skin from becoming dried out during exposure to the elements.

After the age of about 25, even a normal skin loses some of its natural elasticity, so extra care is needed around the vulnerable eye areas. Use a very light eye cream or eye oil at night, patted on sparingly with the tips of the index fingers. Never drag this skin. Although lines will come, this treatment will help to slow down the aging process and soften any existing lines at the same time.

Dry skin *Cleanse* with a rich cleansing cream specially formulated for dry skins. Apply generously to throat, cheeks, forehead and nose. Massage in with light fingertip strokes, then remove with cotton wool [cotton]. Repeat. Use an oily eye make-up remover, very sparingly and lightly (two very light applications are better that one heavy one) and remove with cotton wool [cotton].

Follow this routine night and morning (excluding eye make-up removing process). Avoid using tap water on your face. If you feel you must cleanse your face with water once a day, use mineral water and a creamy face-wash instead of soap.

Tone with a very delicate and light preparation. Possibly one of the best is rose-water diluted with mineral water. This is necessary to remove the last traces of greasy cleanser before putting on moisturizer and make-up. Apply gently on cotton wool [cotton], avoiding the eye and upper cheek area completely.

Moisturize with two kinds of cream: a light, yet nourishing cream for day, and a heavier cream for night. It is possible to buy a very rich moisturizing night cream for dry skins which still disappears rapidly into the pores, so that you don't have to go to bed with a greasy face.

Use a special throat moisturizing cream once a day. Dry skin wrinkles more quickly in the delicate throat area, so you do need to use the moisturizer even in your early twenties. Every night, apply a light under-eye cream with the pads of your index fingers in very gentle movements. Once or twice a week, treat your skin to a moisturizing facial: a good one can be made very simply by mashing the flesh of a ripe avocado pear with a little glycerine or lanolin and applying the mixture to the skin. It should be wiped off gently with damp cotton wool [cotton] after 10 minutes.

Oily skin *Cleanse* twice or even three times a day if you can. It is important to control the oil secretions from the sebaceous glands, and although this is primarily an internal problem (diet adjustment helps), the greasy build-up on the surface of the skin must be removed externally. Use a liquid or medicated skin cleanser and apply generously to the throat, chin, forehead and nose. Dab a little cleanser on each side of your nose, where the oiliness is usually worst. Massage in

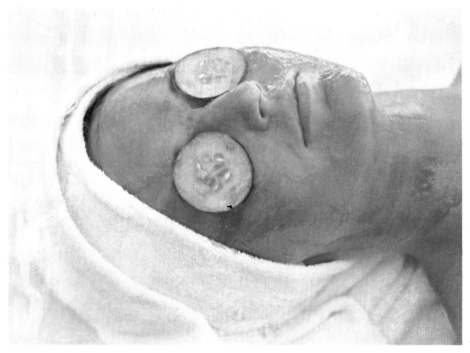

thoroughly, then remove with cotton wool [cotton]. Repeat. If your skin is badly blemished, use a medicated liquid soap with water after this routine.

Tone with an astringent lotion, applying particularly thoroughly to the oiliest places such as sides of the nose, chin and forehead. This will help to close the pores and discourage the greasy excretions from building up too rapidly underneath your make-up. Remember: wearing make-up is actually a protection for your skin. When blemishes occur, it is good for your self-confidence to cover them. It will certainly not make them any worse, as long as a thorough skin cleansing routine is carried out every day.

Moisturize with a light, liquid moisturizer applied sparingly. Even oily skin needs moisturizing for protection and for softening the skin. However, use the moisturizer only once a day — in the morning before making up, or when make-up is reapplied in the evening. At night, follow the toning routine with the application of a little medicated blemish stick on any spots [blemishes]. Never over dry your skin by using harsh antiseptic creams all over your face. You will simply dry off the top layer of skin, leaving the cause of the spots undealt with.

Combination skin *Cleanse* with a light cream, paying particular attention to the greasy areas — nose, chin, forehead. Apply in blobs, massage in lightly with finger tips, then wipe off carefully with cotton wool [cotton]. Repeat. Now use a medicated liquid soap cleanser with water on greasy areas only. Pat dry lightly with a soft

Cucumber contains a natural soothing juice which can liven up tired eyes. Just place a slice on each eye and relax for 10 minutes. Pound the cucumber flesh and mix with a little milk to make a softening facial mask for toning to use while you rest

towel. Follow this routine every night and morning and supplement the basic daily cleansing with a twice-weekly deep cleanse for the particularly greasy areas. Apply a cleansing mask or face pack very carefully to the nose, chin and forehead. Leave this on for about 15 minutes and remove with cotton wool soaked in tepid water.

Tone with a very light toning lotion all over the face, except for the eye area. Next, apply astringent to the greasy areas with cotton wool [cotton]. Never let the astringent go over the dry cheek and eye areas.

Moisturize with liquid moisturizer all over the face, then apply a nourishing moisturizer cream to cheeks only. At night, use a skin food on the dry skin areas. Apply a medicated blemish stick to any spots [blemishes] on chin, nose or forehead. This may seem rather complicated at first, but you will soon become accustomed to the routine. Occasionally, apply neck care cream to your neck. Every night, use a light under-eye cream applied with a very light touch indeed. If the skin over the cheekbone looks rough and flaky, use a nourishing face pack (the one made from avocado flesh described in the Dry Skin section above, for example) on these areas only. Always consider your skin in two sections — dry and greasy.

hands and nails

The hands are one of the hardest-worked parts of the body and they deserve special care. Lovely hands, polished nails and feet with soft skin are as important a part of your beauty as your face and hair.

Care for your hands

Your hands show — at work, at home, when you are travelling, shopping, cooking or simply talking. They are on display. If you work with your hands they need special care so that they both look good and function well. Start with one golden rule: apply a good lubricating hand cream after every rough job and *always* after washing. Choose a hand cream which is absorbed rapidly into the skin and rub it in with firm, smooth strokes — sparing some cream for your forearms and elbows. Treat special problems as soon as they arise.

Hand problems

Roughness and redness occur when natural oils are removed from the skin. Wear rubber gloves for washing up and for the tough and messy household jobs like peeling vegetables. Sprinkle talcum powder inside the gloves before you put them on to keep them fresh-smelling. If water seeps into the gloves, dry them thoroughly before you wear them again. If rubber gloves are too bulky to wear for some jobs, use cotton ones instead. Avoid direct contact with chemical cleansers such as scouring powder, lavatory cleanser, detergents and metal polishes.

If your hands have become rough and sore, try this remedy: cover them with a mixture of 2 tablespoons almond oil, 1 teaspoon honey and the yolk of an egg. Put on cotton gloves for an hour or so, then remove the gloves and wash your hands in a mixture of 1 tablespoon cider vinegar and 1 pint of water. Out of doors in cold weather, wear gloves or mitts in a natural fibre such as wool, and exercise your hands as much as possible. Here are some simple exercise routines:

1 Play a scale, as you would on a piano, on a table surface, using the fingers of each hand alternately.

2 Take the fingers of one hand in the other and gently pull each one of them. (Do this for the fingers of both hands.)

3 Bend the fingers up and down in graceful slow movements.

Eczema A severe hand condition, and it can occur on the arms and other parts of the body, too. You should consult your doctor if you think that you may have eczema. One of the things he may suggest is that you increase the amount of Vitamin B in your diet. You can easily do this by eating liver at least once a week, and by sprinkling wheatgerm over your breakfast cereal. Eczema can be a nervous condition or the result of an allergy, so it is essential to ask the help of a doctor in dealing with it.

Chilblains Caused by bad circulation. Avoid exposing your hands to sudden changes of temperature. Wear gloves with soft thin wool linings in winter and do exercises for suppleness daily. Always dry your hands thoroughly after washing them: dampness can make the chilblains worse.

Clammy hands Usually a nervous condition. Sudden increase in tension can make the eccrine sweat glands in the palms of hands secrete a 'cold sweat'. Keep a stock of cologne-impregnated pads in your handbag and use them to refresh your palms when necessary. Wash regularly with a fresh-smelling soap such as a herbal one.

Allergies A common problem, particularly for people who work with chemicals (hairdressers, lab workers). Sudden contact with a new household product— even something quite mild-sounding like a shampoo or washing powder — can cause an allergic rash to form. Many people are allergic to the enzyme ingredient in some detergents. Metal allergy is also quite common: an irritating, sore patch can form underneath a ring or a bracelet. Remove the metal ornament at once, otherwise the sores could become very painful. (Luckily few women are allergic to gold!)

Nails

Nails are formed by very tightly-packed skin cells which grow from roots in the dermis skin layer. The hard substance formed by these skin cells is called keratin, a version of the substance that makes up the hairs on the head. Keratin is largely formed from calcium and protein, so a diet that includes these things in the shape of meat, fish, cheese, eggs, milk and cream can help to build healthy nails. Unfortunately, most of us subject our nails to a great deal of hard work—cooking, gardening, washing up, typing and so on and they tend to break quickly. About 90 percent of all women suffer from splitting, tearing, soft or brittle nails.

Problem nails

These can be improved with special care. First, check your diet and see that it includes a good supply of the foods mentioned above.

Next, check the hazards which your nails are exposed to.

Gloves If you are breaking your nails while doing housework, try wearing cotton or rubber gloves for some of the tougher jobs.

Types of polish Avoid using pearlized nail polishes if your nails flake or split. These polishes contain fish scales which have a far more drying effect than ordinary cream polishes. Choose the cream polishes if your nails need special care, using a strengthener under the nail colour to give protection. At least one firm now produces nail strengthener in colours, so you can combine protection with a pretty look easily.

When one coat of polish gets chipped remove it completely. Always be sure to do this at least once a week. A build-up of several coats of nail polish can make nails even more dry and flaky. White patches on the nails can result from a calcium deficiency, so increase the milk, cheese and yogurt in your diet.

Filing Be especially careful when filing brittle nails. Use a new emery board, not a worn metal nail file and file the nails in one direction only, not backwards and forwards in a 'sawing' motion, which can easily tear the delicate keratin layers.

Cuticles Use a nourishing cuticle cream when you do your weekly mani-

Three techniques of nail polish application 1. whole nail covered, with tip of nail wiped to leave white 2. half-moon exposed 3. paler top coat brushed over centre of the polished nail to make broad nail appear slimmer

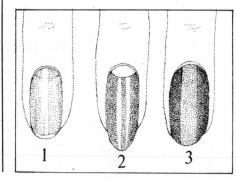

cure, pushing the cuticles well back from the nails. Trim away any jagged piece of hard skin from the edge of the nails with small, sharp nail scissors. Always clean beneath nails thoroughly, using a piece of cotton wool [cotton] on an orange stick. (See the step-by-step manicure section which follows.)

Step-by-step Manicure

Items needed: Nail polish remover; cotton wool [cotton]; bowl of soapy water (do *not* use detergent); cuticle cream; orange sticks; emery boards; base-coat; nail polish.

Step 1 Remove any old nail polish, using a small piece of cotton wool [cotton] and nail polish remover. Always hold the cotton wool [cotton] between the first two joints of the first and second fingers and stroke the nails on the cotton wool [cotton], rather than the other way round. This prevents polish from staining your fingers and the nail polish remover from touching other nails.

Step 2 Cut nails if necessary. File into rounded shape with an emery board. Do not file nails too hard at the sides as this will make them more fragile. Hold the emery board at the narrow end, and always file in the same direction: away from you and not towards you.

Step 3 Put a small blob of cuticle cream on each nail in turn, where the cuticle joins the nail. Massage well into the cuticle to soften it. Ease cuticle back gently from the nail with the edge-shaped end of an orange stick.

Step 4 Dabble nails in soapy water to cleanse them. Remove all traces of dirt and grease from under each nail with the pointed end of an orange stick.

Step 5 Apply nail polish remover again to each nail, holding cotton wool [cotton] as described in Step 1. This will remove all traces of grease, leaving a matte surface for the polish.

Step 6 Apply base-coat very carefully. Paint the right-hand nails first, then the left-hand nails. Allow five minutes for the base-coat to dry thoroughly.

Step 7 Apply nail polish in this way: Take the first stroke up the centre of the nail, from the cuticle almost to the nail tip. Now make a crescent-shaped stroke to the left of this central stroke, ending at the tip of the nail. Make another crescent-shaped stroke to the right of the centre stroke, joining the first stroke at the tip of the nail. Even out all the joins at the nail centre with light strokes. Allow at least first minutes for the polish to dry. Apply second coat.

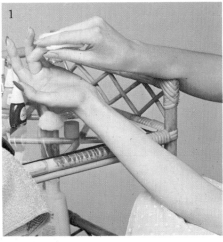
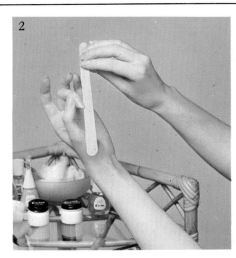
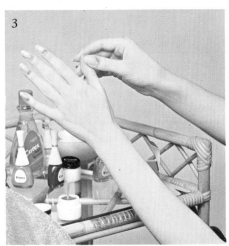
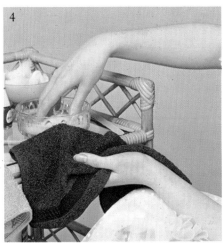
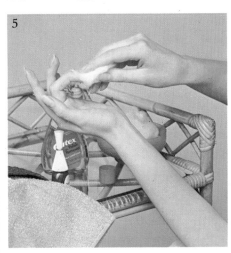
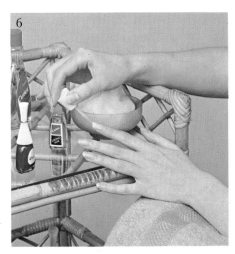
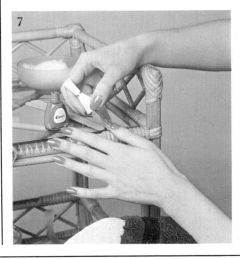
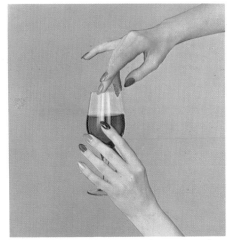

feet & toes

Well-shaped feet are a special beauty asset in summer and a practical asset at any time of the year. Well-cared-for feet help your face to look good too: no one smiles and feels relaxed if her feet are uncomfortable. Look after your feet for the sake of their future, too: foot problems can worsen and even become quite serious in the course of time.

One of the best beauty treatments of all is walking. If your feet aren't up to the effort, you miss out on enjoyable and valuable exercise.

So, examine your feet carefully at least once a week for possible problems. If they start to hurt make absolutely sure that the shoes you are wearing are the right size, sufficiently roomy and giving plenty of arch support. Don't be a slave to fashion if it means spoiling your feet and being uncomfortable. Buy a modified version of the latest fashionable shape which gives you no discomfort.

Foot problems

Beautiful feet are free of sore corns, hard skin and other foot troubles. Here is a list of the most common ones and what to do about them:

Corns are caused by friction and pressure. Shoes that are ill-fitting are often the culprits. The skin becomes compressed and forms a lump which sometimes has a hard central core. The corn may be on the outside of the toe, or between two toes, where it can be particularly painful. It is also liable to turn septic through the moisture trapped between the toes, since germs thrive in the damp warmth.

Do not try to deal with a corn yourself—you'll probably make it worse and far more sore. Visit a chiropodist, who will remove it painlessly. After that set about tackling the cause yourself. Examine your shoes, slippers, tights. Be ruthless about throwing out any that are too tight, (One-size tights which are not large enough can cause constriction.)

Callouses are fairly flat growths with no central core. They are compressed layers of skin that have grown protec-tively over friction-prone areas. The balls of the feet, ankles, heels, under the toes are often affected. They're harder and more painful than simple hard skin and may even be triggered off by some internal bodily upset. See your doctor or chiropodist.

In-growing toe nails are most often caused by bad toenail trimming. Toe nails should always be cut straight across. If they're rounded (like finger nails), the sides of the nails tend to grow up into the soft flesh at the sides of the toes. Inflamed skin is the first sign of an ingrowing toe nail. Get your doctor to treat it without delay, other-wise an infection may start and an operation become necessary. The skin on the ingrown nail will be gently eased back and the nail itself dug out with a sterile probe under strictly antiseptic conditions. The removal of the nail hurts, and sometimes a local or a general anaesthetic is necessary.

Verrucae, which look like warts, are a brown colour and rough to the touch. They are caused by infection commonly found in damp, warm places where people go barefoot (swimming baths, gyms and communal showers). They are particularly painful at the first movement of the foot in the morning. They spread rapidly, so if you find that you have one or two, avoid the probable source of contact and see your doctor or chiropodist for treatment immediately.

Bunions are misaligned joints which become swollen and tender when they are subjected to pressure. Ill-fitting shoes are the likely villains but the underlying cause of the badly-position-ed joint could be hereditary. The bone which joins the big toe to the main arch of the foot is particularly likely to get out of alignment. Bunions are becoming rarer now that shoes are less constricting across the ball of the foot. The soreness they cause can be relieved by careful choice of footwear, or the bunions themselves can be removed altogether by surgery.

Athlete's foot is a fungoid growth caused by a germ which thrives in warm, damp conditions, like those in showers, for example. The woolly socks and the shoes (or boots) worn by people who play tennis, badminton, squash, cricket and football can en-courage the condition — hence its name. The fungus, which is a greyish red in colour and looks like a group of flattened warts, usually feels very itchy and uncomfortable. Consult your doctor or chiropodist if you think that you have athlete's foot. It can be healed by dressings, but it is more usually dealt with surgically.

Foot beauty care

Foot freshness Whenever you bathe, spare a little time for your feet. Cut toe nails as soon as they need it. Trim them straight across to prevent ingrowing nails with sharp scissors or clippers. Next, clean all round the nail area using an orange stick with the tip wrapped in cotton wool [cotton]. This is vital if you've been going about without tights or wearing toeless shoes: dirt tends to col-lect at the sides of the nails particularly. Lavish plenty of body lotion on your feet after you have removed dead skin with pumice. Look for whiskers of hair round your ankle bone and on your toes — they can easily be missed when you are defuzzing your legs. Freshen your feet with deodorant talc, sprinkling this in your shoes too or use a refreshing foot spray. On a really hot day, try paddling tired feet in cold salted water. A foot bath in diluted cider vinegar is also refresh-ing, and it helps remove any itchiness. Make sure that your shoes and tights smell sweet, too. Wash tights every day, and sprinkle talc in your shoes before you put them away. If feet perspire excessively in summer, try going without tights, since the nylon causes a perspiration build-up which would otherwise evaporate quickly. Use an overnight tanning preparation if your feet and legs look too pale.

Exercises Spare some time too for foot and ankle exercises (see right) if you like to wear high heels.

Warm feet

If you have cold feet in bed, massage them at bedtime with a little olive oil, rubbing it in well between your toes. Don't refuse the help of bedsocks, either: warm feet are important.

Shoes Always choose shoes which support the arch well and have plenty of room in the toes. When you come home after a busy day and slip thank-fully out of your shoes, do not put on a pair of flat, fluffy bedroom slippers. Instead, change into com-fortable shoes — perhaps ones that are slightly out of fashion now. Beware of clog-type wooden exercise sandals with a strap across the instep. Chiropo-dists point out that these can only be beneficial if the wooden sole clog corresponds exactly in shape to the sole of your feet. Since these clogs are mass-produced to one shape only, the chances are that you may be spoiling your feet by wearing them.

Exercises for feet and ankles

1 Keep heel firmly on floor, raise toes and instep and twist them gently but strongly outwards. Do this exercise for both feet in any odd moments — when you are sitting on a train or at a desk or waiting for someone.

2 Move toes firmly up and down, 10 times for each foot.

Step-by-step Pedicure

Items needed: Toenail clippers; orange sticks; cuticle cream; small pieces of sponge or cotton wool [cotton]; polish remover; base coat; nail polish.

Step 1 Remove any old nail polish, using cotton wool [cotton] and a little nail polish remover. Hold the cotton wool [cotton] between the first two joints of the first and second finger. In this way you will avoid removing your finger-nail polish as you work. Trim nails with nail clippers. Cut nails straight across, not rounded or pointed.

Step 2 File nails gently. Use the rougher side of the emery board first, then the finer side to give a smooth finish. Hold the narrow end of the board and grasp each toe in turn.

Step 3 Put a blob of cuticle cream on each nail in turn, and massage gently into the cuticle. Using the wedge-shaped end of an orange stick, gently ease back the cuticles. Put a little cuticle remover on cotton wool [cotton], wrapped around the pointed end of the orange stick. Ease away dirt and loose skin from beneath each toenail and from the sides of the nail.

Step 4 Dabble toes in a little soapy water. Massage dry gently with a towel. Use a little body lotion to soften hard skin on your feet. Do not smear this lotion over your toes. It would put a greasy surface on the nails and make the polish difficult to apply.

Step 5 Apply base-coat — or clear nail polish used as a base-coat — to each toe. Hold the toe gently between forefinger and thumb as you work.

Step 6 Place small pieces of sponge or cotton wool [cotton] between the toes of your right foot. Hold the ball of your foot in your left hand, with the thumb resting lightly just above the toes. Apply the polish carefully with three distinct strokes for each nail: first, up the centre of the nail, next, on the left of the centre stroke and third, on the right of the centre stroke. Always paint away from yourself and do not have too much polish on the brush for each stroke. Repeat the process on the left foot. Allow polish to dry for at least five minutes. Apply second coat.

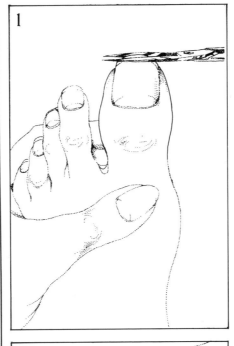

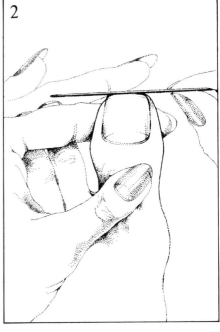

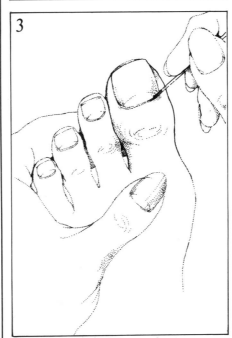

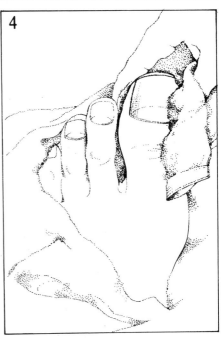

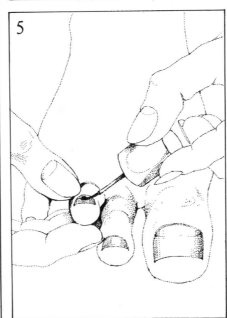

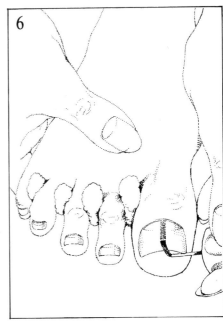

keeping smooth

Unwanted and unnecessary hair can be one of the most embarrassing beauty problems. Fortunately, methods of dealing with it have become so common in beauty salons all over the world, that women are now prepared to discuss it openly. Few women have to cope with the problem of a bristly moustache or shaggy growth on their legs, but almost everyone has some unwanted body hair. Here is a list of the various kinds of body hair and the best methods for dealing with each kind.

Underarm hair

If underarm hair is left alone, it provides additional coverage and warmth for the rapid growth and multiplication of the bacteria which cause underarm odour. Therefore, it is necessary for the sake of basic hygiene to remove it quite apart from the fact that it looks unsightly. This hair grows quickly, so it needs tackling at least twice a week.

Shaving Quickest for the underarm, since it can be easily incorporated into your beauty routine. However, you must use a ladies' razor — a sharp one — with considerable care and do the shaving in front of a mirror so that you don't miss any crevices. (An electric razor is a very good buy for this purpose.) After soaping and shaving, dust the underarms with talc. Deodorize much later in the day since any anti-perspirant preparation will sting sharply and painfully on just-shaved skin.

Depilatory creams Another good method for removing underarm hair. The disadvantage for busy people is that it is necessary to wait for about five minutes while the cream 'melts' away the hair. Then the cream must be removed with a wooden spatula. However, depilatory cream gives a slightly smoother finish than shaving and the results last a little longer, because the hair is dissolved just below the skin's surface.

Some women find that shaving works well as a regular routine, supplemented by the use of a depilatory cream when a really smooth finish is required — in summer, for example, or just before going out in a sleeveless dress.

Waxing is sometimes used for the underarm area when long lasting smoothness is required — just before

a holiday, for instance. (The results of waxing last about five weeks.) However, waxing is painful in this particular area, and should be done by an expert. You might give up halfway through if you tried it yourself!

Facial hair

This is caused by hormonal imbalance. Many women find that one or two (or more) hairs appear on their face during the menopause. (There is some evidence too that the contraceptive pill causes facial hair to grow.) The male hormones which are causing the growth of hair may cease activity after menopause.

However, some younger women (usually those whose hair is dark) do find that they have an embarrassing dark down on their face, on the upper lip or sides of the face. There are several ways of dealing with this, and the method you choose muse be governed by the amount and type of facial hair.

Plucking Only suitable for isolated hairs on the chin. If you have just one or two coarse black hairs here, plucking them out with eyebrow tweezers when necessary will solve the problem. Don't try to pluck out hairs on the upper lip, however. You'll not only make your face very sore, but you will also make the job of the electrolysist (see section below on Electrolysis) more difficult if you later decide to have the hairs removed professionally.

Bleaching Suitable only for very fine, downy hair. Use a very mild solution of peroxide and water and try it on the down on the back of your hand first. If it works there satisfactorily, dab a very little on the offending hairs with cotton wool, protecting the surrounding skin with a tissue.

If you have a few fine, dark hairs straggling downwards from the natural hairline at the side of your face, bleaching may be a solution. It will tend to weaken the existing hair, but the new hair will of course, grow as dark and strong as before. If bleaching is impractical, electrolysis is worth considering, even for fine hair.

Electrolysis A method of cauterizing the hair-root with a tiny electric shock. It's important to choose a highly experienced and qualified electrolysist who belongs to a recognized professional body; someone unskilled could do

a lot of harm. And you must be prepared to allow nine weeks for the whole treatment.

Leg hair

Coarse, dark leg hair is most embarrassing in summer, when swim suits, bikinis and short dresses reveal bare legs. However, it is a good idea, for the sake of your self-confidence, to deal with this hair all the time, and not just at times of year when it shows most. The way you deal with leg hair depends on the coarseness.

Bleaching This works well for fair, downy hair. If the growth is quite short and fine, but just a little too dark for comfort, use a weak solution of peroxide on a little cotton wool every few weeks. In hot weather you will find that the hair growth becomes fairer in the sunshine, so the bleaching process will not be necessary very often. Bleaching weakens the hair, too.

Shaving It has one disadvantage for leg hair. The regrowth is stubbly and rough and it returns too rapidly for comfort! If you have dark leg hairs, the regrowth may also look shadowy and grubby, and consequently very unpleasant. There is the danger, too, of cutting the skin, particularly over the shinbone.

Depilatory creams These give a smooth finish on the legs but must be used twice a week for lasting results. However, the regrowth is not stubbly, so if you miss a day, it is not at all disastrous. Apply the cream all over the hairy area, wait for about five minutes, then remove the cream with a spatula. Next wash or shower in lukewarm water and then rub in some moisturizing cream as the depilatory cream is very drying.

Depilatory creams in aerosol form are more convenient to use. You simply spray on the cream, wait the required five minutes, then remove with a spatula. Wash and moisturize afterwards. The aerosol method is suitable for a medium to dark growth of hair.

Waxing A good answer to the problem of dark, tough hair, as the results last for about five weeks. However, it is fairly painful, so try it first at a beauty salon, not at home.

If the discomfort does not worry you and you decide to do the waxing the next time yourself, it's a good idea to share the chore with a friend. Take great care (1) not to apply the wax too hot and (2) to rip it off in one long continuous tug (or to get your friend to do so). Don't pull a little, then hesitate, then pull some more: it will hurt far more.

Treat yourself to a salon waxing before a holiday, whatever type of leg hair you have: it is marvellous to be able to forget completely about this particular chore for a few weeks.

Electrolysis Not recommended for most types of leg hair, particularly as the scabs take some time to heal. There are about 830 hair follicles to the square inch and even a expert electrolysist can only remove about 300 hairs in a session.

However, if the hair is so thick and black that you have to remove it daily, or even twice a day, then electrolysis may be a good solution. Wearing tights and stockings twists the hair in the follicles, so the electrolysist may have a problem in finding the root with the electrode as she probes. In addition, a stronger current is required for tough leg hair than for softer facial hair. If you think electrolysis may be the best answer to a serious problem consult an expert about it.

Thigh hair

Pubic hair often grows down the inside of the thighs, and when it is dark, it can be very embarrassing if you wear a swimsuit or a bikini. The skin is tender on this area, so you must remove the hair with great care.

Shaving Not recommended for the thighs. The soft skin may become blotchy looking and the regrowth will be stubbly and unattractive. It will show, too.

Depilatory creams These should be used with great care on the thighs. Choose the strength usually recommended for facial hair, since ordinary-strength cream may cause soreness.

Waxing This works well but is painful, and may cause temporary redness. However, it is a good method to use just before a holiday — say three or four days ahead to let the redness subside. Electrolysis is a good, lasting method for this area. However, have the hair removed during the winter, so that the area will have healed thoroughly before you go swimming in summer. Do not be embarrassed about deciding to have electrolysis. There are very many women with the same hair problem and electrolysists are glad to deal with it. Let the hair grow for six weeks before your first appointment.

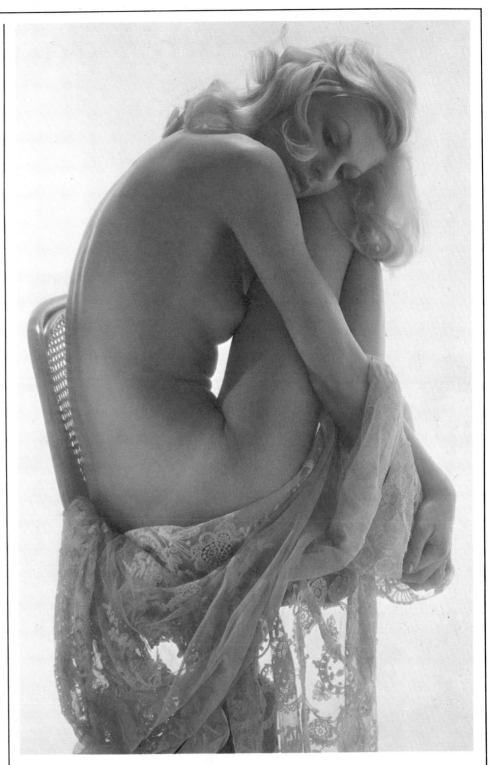

A smooth skin is achieved with regular de-fuzzing and constant beauty care

Breast and stomach hair

Many women have a few hairs growing around their nipples and navels. Some even have a very hairy growth in a stripe between the navel and the pubic area. It is unwise to try to remove hair on the breasts or the stomach yourself by plucking, shaving or depilatory creams.

Electrolysis is the best method and is quite safe for these areas of the body. As always, choose a time for the treatment when you won't be wearing a swimsuit for several months. This will give the tiny scabs time to heal properly.

Hair on the lower back

A small 'tuft' of hair growing on the lower back is very common.

Electrolysis is the best way of getting rid of this hair, for the same reasons as it is for breast and stomach hair. However, if the hair is growing from a birthmark or mole, check with your doctor before making an appointment for electrolysis.

...and don't neglect these patches

Areas for Special Care

Daily care can help keep your whole body smooth and soft. But sometimes specific problems arise which need particular attention. Here are details about improving skin texture, colour and tone.

Neck This can be one of the most neglected areas of the body, yet it is the neck which gives away a woman's age almost before anything else. Include it in all facial beauty routines — cleansing, toning and nourishing.

If you neck is already crepey-looking and covered in fine lines, use a special nourishing cream every night and stimulate circulation with gentle massage, moving your hands alternately from the base of the throat upwards to the chin in a flowing movement.

Upper arms If faulty circulation makes your arms look mottled and unattractive, rub them briskly with a friction mitt when you are in the bath and then rinse with hot and cold water alternatively. Add a little Epsom salts to your bathwater or try a seaweed or peat bath for additional stimulation. (Health stores and some chemists stock the items you need for these.) Beware of sitting with your arms too close to an open fire and of sudden changes in temperature.

If your upper arms are thick, with a tough-looking skin which looks rather like pale orange peel, it may be affected by cellulitis. This condition, usually found on the thighs and stomach, as well as on the upper arms, is caused by an infection of the subcutaneous skin tissues. Very stringent massage can help to break up the deposits of fat. A diet which includes plenty of fresh fruit (particularly oranges and lemons) and green vegetables can help too. Pinch the area in the bath (it won't hurt much) and try a professional massage. Whiteheads, which often appear on the backs of the upper arms, are caused by acidity in the skin. Treat them by patting almond or olive oil on the area, then wrapping it in a hot towel for a few minutes. The skin will soften and the whiteheads will loosen. Extract them with an ordinary blackhead extractor. Ask someone else to do this for you if you find it difficult to reach the backs of your arms.

Elbows Take a look at your elbows. If they are dry, wrinkled and red-looking, give them a beauty treatment every day just by remembering to smooth your handcream up to elbow level each time you use it. Soften elbows and make them whiter by leaning them in

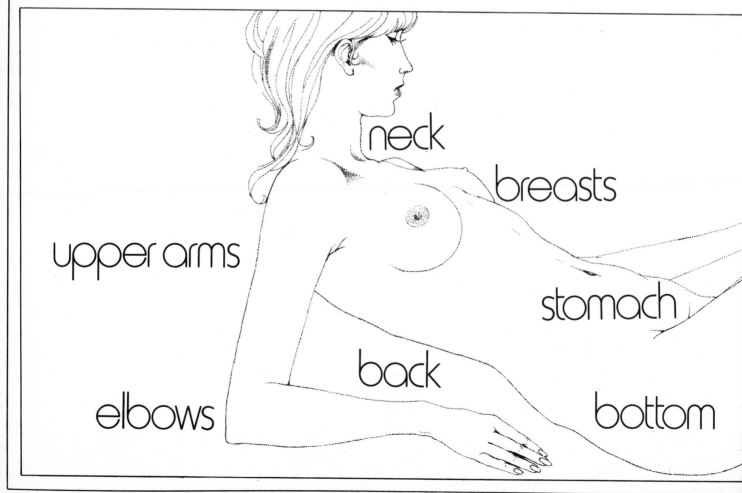

halves of fresh lemon. It's good a idea to keep a lemon, cut in half, by the kitchen sink. Then, whenever you have a moment or two to spare, give your elbows a quick beauty treatment. If they are very sore, apply a soothing paste made from a cup of oatmeal mixed with a little boiling milk. Allow this to cool, smooth it on your elbows and leave it there for a few moments. Then wash it off with lukewarm water.

Stomach Stretch marks here result when the fibres beneath the surface of the skin weaken and the normal, elasticity of skin is not great enough to cope with this. The marks most commonly occur just after childbirth, but they can also appear suddenly in puberty, when the growth rate is very fast. The best cure is prevention — the application of olive or baby oil throughout pregnancy and immediately after the birth of the baby. However, if marks have appeared, lubricating the skin can certainly help to minimize the less severe ones. So can suntan treatments since they help to even up the skin tone. The marks may also fade a little with regular application of a cream containing a large concentration of Vitamin E. More serious stretch marks are difficult to disguise and sometimes surgery may be recommended.

Breasts If you have mottled-looking skin on the breasts, stimulate circulation with alternative rinses of hot and cold water. It will help to minimize the problem and make your bosom firmer. If the skin looks wrinkled and sagging (perhaps after childbirth or breast-feeding), use a good moisturizing cream and follow the exercises in the section called Keeping Fit.

Thighs Thick 'orange peel' skin here is usually caused by cellulitis and needs tough, regular massage by a beautician. Mottled skin on the thighs indicates faulty circulation, and you can improve this with the help of a friction mitt used in circular motion.

Knees Rough, red knees respond to pampering with body lotion and nourishing moisturizing creams. Rub them with baby oil or olive oil after bathing.

Back Spotty backs are often a problem for people who tend to have greasy or combination facial skin.

The spots will be aggravated by contact with greasy hair, so a regular shampoo and/or dandruff treatment is necessary. The over-active sebaceous glands that cause the greasy secretions which start the spots are themselves stimulated by hormonal activity in the body, particularly in adolescence. The only remedy is to keep the skin scrupulously clean by washing with a medicated liquid soap daily and by changing the clothes next to the skin every day. To avoid unnecessary irritation, choose cotton if possible for the vest, bra, blouse or T-shirt which is next to the spotty area. Apply a medicated cleansing lotion and an anti-acne cream to dry up the excess grease at bedtime. If a spot appears on your back just before you plan to wear a low-backed or backless evening dress, disguise it with a medicated made-up stick matching your skin-tone.

Bottom Bottoms are sun- and air-starved. Even in summer, they are kept covered, so no wonder they tend to look pale and pasty. Nude sunbathing is impractical for most of us, but instead of that you can use an ultra-violet lamp for a few seconds every day, or have a course of ultra-violet treatments. Always moisturize this area of your body with plenty of body lotion. If the flesh is bulgy and bumpy, literally pummell it into shape by bumping each cheek against a wall for a count of 10 every day. Pinching the flesh on your bottom when you are in the bath is also good for circulation and shape.

Although bottoms are meant to be sat on, they're not meant to be sat on all the time. Walking provides good bottom-shaping exercise, and 'walking' on your bottom will help to reduce bulges and tone the skin.

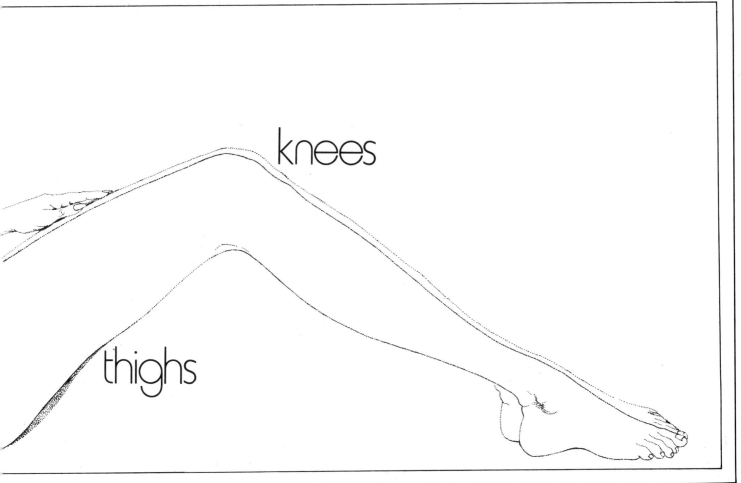

you and the elements

Intense cold and extreme heat can have a bad effect on the skin. Probably the ideal climate for keeping the skin soft and smooth is a mild, wet one. However, in these days of easy travel, even people who generally live in an ideal climate are likely to subject their skins to sudden rises and drops in temperature.

Heat

Heat has a drying, aging effect on all but the most oily of skins. As the natural oils begin to dry, the skin becomes leathery and may wrinkle. The leathery texture and brown pigment are actually the skin's own natural protection against the effect of ultra violet radiation. Extra Vitamin D is produced in the skin when the body is exposed to radiation.

To protect itself against excessive production of this vitamin, and to prevent sunburn, the skin produces melanin — the brown pigment we know as sun-tan — increases the thickness of the epidermis and hastens the keratinization of the outer layer (see Care for Your Skin).

The solution to the aging problem is to replace the lost moisture with all over moisturizing daily and sun tan oils. If the skin is particularly dry or sensitive these should contain an effective sun screen. Because it is fashionable to have a golden tan, many women rush into a tanning programme on the very first day of their holiday, often with disastrous consquences. Remember that a light, gold tone to the skin can be just as attractive as a deep reddish-brown and is far healthier. Consult the chart *right* to find a tanning programme for your skin type.

Another important factor has been discovered that can help to solve the problem of burning. The level of Vitamin A in the blood drops after the body is exposed to intensive ultraviolet radiation, so taking extra Vitamin A just before and during a holiday helps to prevent burning by increasing the thickness of the skin. Stores of Vitamin A in the body are affected too by the extra Vitamin D formed during exposure to the sun. Consequently, taking extra Vitamin A helps to restore the natural balance. A point to remember: the level of Vitamin A in the body drops during menstruation so extra care is needed if you sunbathe at this time.

Cold

Cold also drys and roughens the skin — particularly dry and sensitive types of skin. Sudden exposure to intense cold can produce blotchiness, hasten the appearance of thread veins on the cheeks and give the skin a flaky appearance. Moisturizing and make-up are the best protection in this case. Be especially lavish with moisturizer during cold weather, and never venture out of doors without a good protective layer of foundation on your skin.

Do not subject the skin to sudden extremes of temperature — don't dash in from the snow to sit close to the heat. This may produce scorch marks on arms and legs and cause chilblains.

Salt water

Salt water is generally invigorating and good for the skin if the salt is later removed with a fresh-water shower afterwards. If it is not, the salt will make the skin — particularly facial skin — excessively dry and may produce burning. If you love to swim, remember that the sun's rays can be heightened by reflection on the salt water, even though you may feel cool. Many painful cases of sunburn are produced in this way.

Tap water

Water from the tap can be good for your skin, depending on your skin-type and the hardness or softness of the water itself. If your skin is extemely dry, washing your face in tap water will not be helpful, for the salts and calcium in the water will almost certainly be drying. Use of a water-softener when washing would help to counteract this effect. However, it is probably more practical to use a softening substance such as bath salts or oil for bathing the rest of your body, and to beware of using hard water on your face. For a freshening face-spray in hot weather, mineral water is ideal: put the water in a well-washed spray bottle and direct it straight on to your skin.

Central heating and air conditioning

Both are potential enemies of good skin. In a hot, airless office, where there may be particles of dust and dirt in the atmosphere, even a normally well behaved skin may rebel. Heavy foundation make-up becomes cloggy and if secretions build up underneath, spots result. It is wise to keep make-

Tanning Chart (times refer to length of exposure on each side)

Burns easily Never sunbathe between 12 noon and 2 pm!
Dry skin Sunscreen first few days, then oil or cream. Or, opt out with overnight tan cream. After-sun moisturiser each night. Day 1-3: 5 minutes. Day 4-6: 10 minutes. After: 20 minutes maximum.
Normal skin Oil, cream or spray mousse. After-sun moisturiser each night. Day 1-3: 5 minutes. Day 4-6: 15 minutes. After: gradually add time as tan darkens. Cover red areas for a day or two.
Oily skin Cream or mousse. After-sun moisturiser alternate nights. Day 1-3: 5 minutes. Day 4-6: 15-20 minutes with caution. After: gradually add time.
Normal sensitivity to sun
Dry skin Cream, oil or lotion. After-sun moisturiser each night. Day 1-3: 5-10 minutes. After: 10-20 minutes. Take care when swimming, sight-seeing, etc.
Normal skin Cream, oil or lotion. After-sun moisturiser alternate nights. Day 1-3: 10 minutes. After: 15 minutes, increasing gradually. Watch for burning.
Oily skin Mousse or oil-free lotion. After-sun moisturiser as needed. Day 1-3: 15 minutes. After: Increase gradually for desired depth of tan.
Seldom burns
Dry skin Lotion or mousse. After-sun moisturiser each night. Day 1-3: 15 minutes. After: 20 minutes, increasing gradually. Avoid leathery dryness.
Oily skin Oil-free lotion. Day 1-3: 15 minutes, increasing to 30. After: Increase gradually for desired depth of tan.

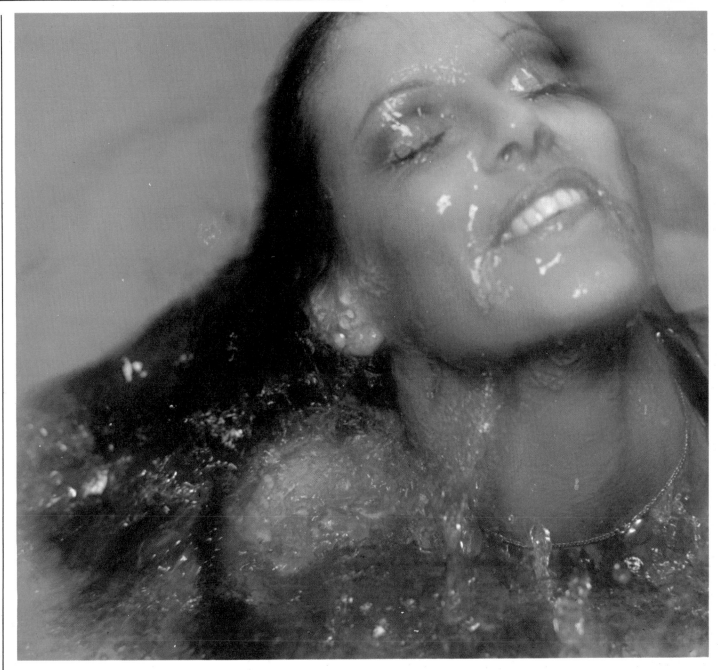

up to a minimum — moisturizer for protection and a light foundation only—and to avoid constant retouching with a cake powder preparation. Deep cleansing every night and the use of a cleansing masque at least once a week will help to keep the skin fresh.

Waterproof make-up

If you love to swim or go surf-riding, there is no need to return to the dry land with smudged and messy make-up. **Eye make-up** Today most manufacturers make waterproof mascara and there are some waterproof eye shadows, too. Waterproof eye make-up must always be removed with the utmost care, with an oily solvent made for that particular product. Do not try to scrub away waterproof eye make-up with soap and water: you will pull your eye lashes out in the process!

Lipstick Non-smudging (indelible) lipsticks have been available for years. Unfortunately, although the colour may stay put, the lipsticks do not give a shiny look to the mouth: A tinted lipgloss is probably the best choice of lip make-up for swimming and sunning. **Foundation and moisturizer** In summer, the lightest touch of make-up is most flattering, especially if the skin is tanned. But salt water has a very drying effect on the skin, so plenty of moisturizer on your face is necessary. A tan-coloured foundation can act as a protection for the most vulnerable parts of your face (nose and forehead, for instance). If this is blended carefully into the skin it will survive the effects of sea water very well. **Eye brows** Always try to keep eye brows well-shaped on holiday. Eye

If you love to swim, but hate looking un-made-up, look for the new waterproof eye shadows, eye liners, mascara and lipsticks. Bright, glowing colours look marvellous with a tan-stunning against green water, blue sky and yellow sand. But make sure you protect your skin with a moisturizing sun-tan lotion—eyelids, cheekbones, neck and forehead are particularly vulnerable

pencil does not stand up to sea-water, so it is best to rely on the shape of the brows themselves for effect. If the brow hairs are very light, it may be advisable to have them dyed a little darker before you go on holiday. If you decide to do this, remember that your eye lashes may need dyeing too. Make an appointment in good time with a beauty salon.

keeping fresh

You may be confident that you smell fresh and sweet at all times of the day, but you can't be sure unless you follow a regular daily freshness routine. The last person to realize that she or he has a 'B.O.' problem is usually the sufferer!

Perspiration

This is simply the product of a continuous cooling process which is absolutely necessary to a healthy existence. It is secreted by over 2 million sweat glands all over the body. There are two types: the eccrine glands (particularly on the hands and the soles of feet) which produce sweat fairly continuously in an almost clear form (about 99 per cent water, 1 per cent sodium and other salts), and the appocrine glands in the underarm and pubic regions. These secrete a milky fluid which decomposes fast to form a breeding ground for bacteria. Although the perspiration secreted by the eccrine glands has no smell in itself, it attracts the bacteria bred by the stale appocrine type of sweat. The amount of perspiration is increased by an increase in warmth and also by emotional changes in the body. Unfortunately, these changes provoke the appocrine glands to work, and this is the perspiration that forms odour.

Deodorants and anti-perspirants

Most people need to use some kind of deodorant or anti-perspirant. Perspiration is often trapped by clothing (particularly in the non-porous, man-made fibres) and the unpleasantness of its smell is increased. Most products now contain an anti-perspirant which will actually stop the glands in a particular area from secreting perspiration at all. The body quickly adapts to this situation and secretes extra perspiration somewhere else more convenient — on the legs, for instance, instead of under the arms. The ingredient in the anti-perspiration product is almost always some kind of aluminium salt substance. People who are allergic to it should take extra care to wash frequently and to use a simple deodorant product which perfumes the smell of sweat rather than stopping it from forming.

In rare cases, this is not a satisfactory solution, and a doctor may recommend a surgical operation to remove the underarm sweat glands entirely. However, this operation is still not widely available.

The daily freshness routine

All-over freshness Have a bath, a shower or an all-over wash every morning. Perspiration builds up in a warm bed and, if you neglect that daily wash it may just be reaching the decomposition stage when you start the day. (See Beauty and the Bath.)

Pay special attention to underarm and pubic areas when you are washing, and use a deodorant soap if possible. In hot weather, or if you perspire a great deal a twice-daily, all-over wash is necessary.

Dry yourself carefully, then apply *deodorant or anti-perspirant* to the underarm area. Probably the most effective kind of anti-perspirant is the roll-on kind: it reaches every part of the cosy underarm hollow and contains more active ingredients than other types. A roll-on deodorant is also the most economical, since there's far less wastage with it.

Now apply *vaginal deodorant*. This should be done carefully and only if you feel that you need it — during a menstrual period, for instance. It can be dangerous to apply too much deodorant too close to the vagina. Some natural secretions in this area of the body are perfectly usual — indeed, they form a protection against infection. However, if they become embarrassing, either in smell or quantity, do not try to deal with them with a deodorant. Consult your doctor.

Allow the deodorant or anti-persipirant to dry thoroughly before putting on your clothes. If you don't, you will simply wipe it away on to your clothes, and that may cause staining. If possible make sure that the garment next to your skin is made of cool, porous cotton, so that perspiration will escape easily, rather than being 'dammed up' by a non-porous fabric. A cotton bra and vest, as well as cotton panties, are the best choice. If you are much troubled by perspiration, try to choose natural fibres for your top garments,

too: bra, sweater, dress, skirt or trousers — and wear stockings rather than nylon tights.

During the day, check underarms for wetness and apply a freshening pad impregnated with anti-perspirant or a little deodorant talc at least once.

At night, wash underarms and pubic area, even if there is no time for a second all-over wash or a bath.

Feet and hands In summer, keep feet sweet-smelling by using a special *deodorant foot spray* daily and by sprinkling a little deodorant talc in your tights and shoes. It may be necessary to do this in the winter too if your feet tend to perspire in a centrally-heated office or home, or if you like to wear snug, close-fitting shoes or boots. Always wash tights or socks daily.

If your hands often become clammy and sweaty through emotional or nervous tension, then keep *cologne-impregnated pads* in your handbag and wipe them often, even when it's not possible to go and wash them thoroughly. Make sure that your gloves are made of natural fibres — leather, wool or cotton.

Caring for clothing If perspiration (or your anti-perspirant) stains your clothing, soak the garment in a solution of soap flakes or liquid soap overnight, and wash it thoroughly the next day. Sponge non-washable fabrics with soap and water or point out the stain to your dry cleaner. If the mark will not budge, dye the garment or discard it.

Cotton dress-shields can protect clothing against excessive perspiration effectively, but they must be washed regularly. Once a garment is really spoilt by perspiration, it is best to throw it away, for the marks are very unsightly.

Never wear a blouse or sweater more than once or, at most, twice before it is washed and change your panties daily. Beware of pulling on a dark-coloured sweater day after day without really thinking about its cleanliness. You may not notice the odour that has built up in the garment, simply because it doesn't look dirty, but other people will be aware of it.

Underarm hair Remove underarm hair (see Keeping Smooth) as it does provide a warm haven for active bacteria.

keeping fit

A beautiful body should be lithe and supple. Many people lead a sedentary life nowadays, and so some form of daily exercise routine is necessary to keep the body in shape. The following six exercises are designed to be followed daily — *regular* exercise is the only really effective form of exercise.

1 Waist, midriff
Stand straight, feet 12 inches apart, left hand by your side and right arm extended above your head with the elbow bent. Keeping your back straight, bend sideways from your waist to the left, sliding your left arm down your leg as you go. Go as far as you can comfortably, straighten up, and repeat to the right 3 times each.

2 Bust
Stand straight, feet 12 inches apart, arms by your sides. Now make large circles backwards in a windmill action, one arm following the other and both moving at the same speed.

3 Stomach
Lie on the floor, hands by your sides, with knees bent and toes tucked securely under the bottom edge of a piece of heavy furniture. Now sit up slowly, taking the strain on your stomach muscles. Lower your body slowly and relax.

4 Thighs
Lie on your left side on the floor, legs straight, one arm resting comfortably on the floor in front of you, the other stretched out under your head. Now raise your right leg as high as you can, hold the position briefly, and lower. Roll over on the right side and repeat with your left leg.

5 Bottom
Sit on your heels with back perfectly straight, hands clasped above your head with elbows bent slightly. Move slowly into a kneeling position and lower bottom to touch the floor to the right of your heels. Hold the position briefly, then rise to a kneeling position once more. Lower your bottom to touch the floor to the left of your heels. Return to starting position.

6 Knees, calves, posture and tone
Stand straight with feet together and back straight. Place your hands on your waist. Now bend knees slowly and descend to a crouching position without wobbling and without bending your back. Hold position briefly, then rise slowly to starting position.

Facial exercises
The object of doing facial exercises is to improve and strengthen muscle tone and to increase blood circulation. Repeat each exercise 10 times.

Double chin (a)
Sit straight, facing a mirror. Now look up to the ceiling, stretching your neck as you do so. Still in the 'stretched upwards' position, turn your head to look over your left shoulder. Return to front, then look over your right shoulder. Return to front, and lower chin to right-angle position with neck.

Flabby jawline (b)
Sit straight, facing a mirror. Clench teeth hard and curl back lips. Stretch corners of your mouth as far apart as you can in a 'grimace' expression. Hold the contraction for a count of six, then relax. Thrust lower jaw as far forward as you can, then relax.

Fat cheeks (c)
Sit straight, facing a mirror. Suck in cheeks, then blow them out alternately. Now 'smile' with one side of your mouth only, pushing the half-grin up and out. Repeat with the other side of your mouth.

Furrowed brow (d)
Sit straight, facing a mirror. Open eyes wide and raise eyebrows at the same time. Hold briefly. Lower brows, bringing eyes back to normal size as you do.

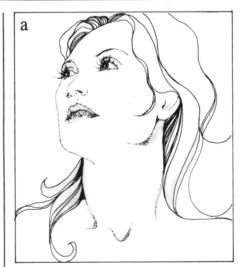

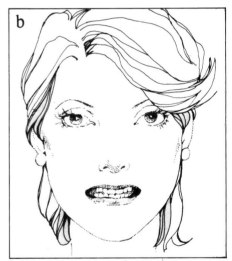

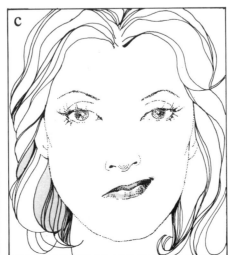

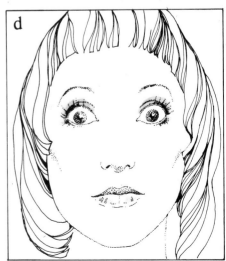

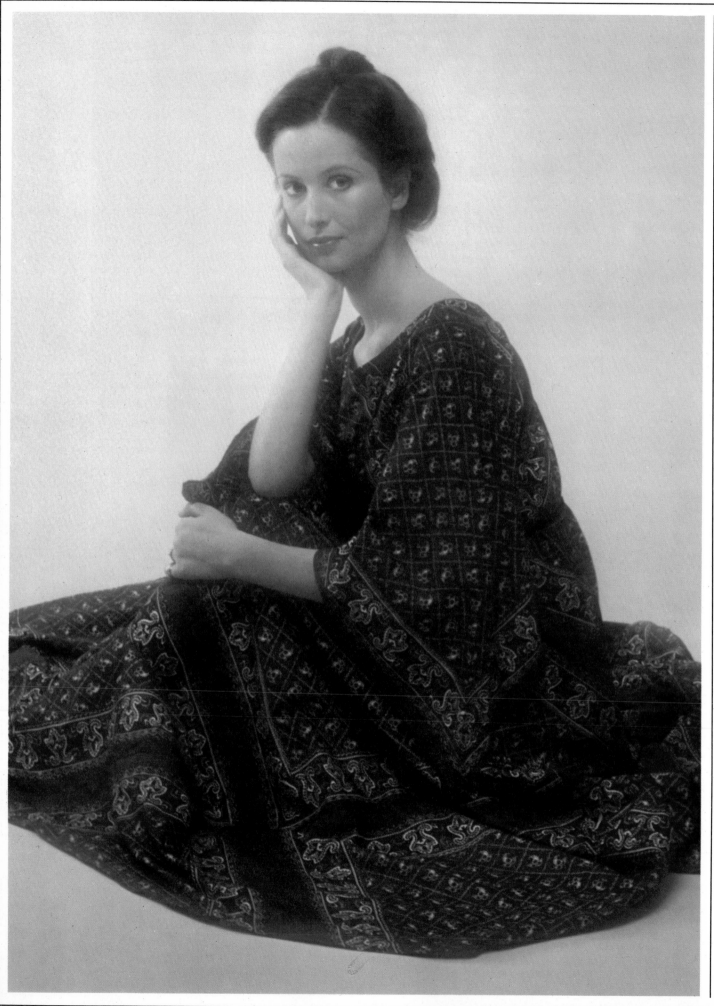

beauty in motion

Beauty in a woman is the sum total of her looks, and the way she moves and her general posture. A slouching walk, an inelegant sitting position, can easily spoil the looks of someone who is otherwise very attractive. One of the most candid tests is to catch sight of yourself suddenly, reflected in a shop window. Is that woman with the drooping shoulders, the jerky walk and the worried frown on her face really you? It can be quite a shock!

The way to perfect beauty in motion is to practise good posture, an elegant walk and a graceful sitting position consciously until they become a spontaneous part of your way of life. It helps, too, to join a movement or keep-fit class or to take up dancing, ice-skating or gymnastics. Avoid hurried, jerky gestures, which are ugly as well as uneconomical in terms of the energy used, at all times. Even if you have to run for a train, you can learn to do it gracefully.

Correct standing posture

Good posture is a health asset as well as a beauty asset. If the shoulders sag forward, the chest will be cramped and lungs will not be able to expand properly. The cells of the body will not obtain enough oxygen, and the result could be fatigue and lack of energy. If the backbone curves too much, the stomach and intestines will be cramped and digestive problems could result. Stand like this:

1 Stretch the body upwards and hold it comfortably — not stiffly — with the weight evenly distributed on both feet
2 Hold the hip girdle evenly, with both sides at the same level
3 Contract the buttock muscles slightly, and hold the stomach in
4 Keep shoulders down and back a little, but not forced into an unnatural position
5 Hold the arms loosely by the sides. If you are standing correctly, an imaginary straight line drawn from the ear to the ground should pass through the neck, shoulder joint, elbow, hand, hip joint, knee and front of the ankle. Practise this posture when you are forced to stand still anywhere for several minutes.

Correct walking posture

Walking gracefully will help to make you look slimmer and more attractive. It will help to show off your clothes to advantage, too.

1 The basic position should be as described in the correct standing posture procedure above
2 The weight of the body should be tilted forward as the weight is switched from the back to the front foot
3 Toes should always point directly forward, not outwards or inwards
4 The arms should swing slightly to and fro, but not in an exaggerated way
5 The hips should be level, not swinging from side to side. Practise this posture as you walk. Check up on your progress from time to time glancing at your reflection in shop windows.

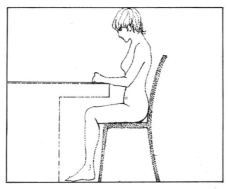

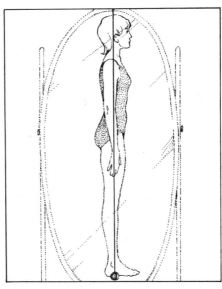

*Top: always sit correctly as you work
Below: hang a piece of weighted twine
from the top of your mirror as a guide*

Correct sitting posture

Here is the correct way to sit on a hard chair, when you are working at a desk for instance.

1 Check that the chair and desk are the correct height. If you work in the same office every day, it makes sense to be comfortable
2 Sit with bottom pressed against the back of the chair, thighs evenly pressed down on the seat, with the hip joint forming a right angle
3 Rest feet flat on the floor with the knee and ankle joints forming right angles
4 Hold shoulders back a little and keep the backbone upright in its natural curves.

Everyday movements

Think how you can move most gracefully in everyday situations. For instance:

Bending down to pick up an object from the floor is more comfortable and looks better if you bend from the knees instead of bending over from the hips. If necessary, hold a table top or chair lightly for balance as you go down.

Stretching upwards to reach something on a high shelf looks best if you stand on the balls of both feet instead of wobbling dangerously and inelegantly on one.

Climbing out of a car seat (particularly a low one) looks ugly if arms and legs are sprawled. Keep knees together, bend legs and swing them out in one movement, holding the car seat for balance. When getting into the car seat, sit down first then bring knees together, tuck up legs and swing into the car.

Sitting on a deep armchair or sofa can be difficult if you don't know quite how soft or resilient the upholstery is. Lower yourself gradually, holding the arm or back of the sofa for balance. Then ease your bottom into the chair when you have safely made contact with the seat. To get up, ease yourself towards the front of the chair first, then stand up. Do not try to haul yourself up from a comfortable, sunken position in one movement. You won't be able to make it!

inner health, outer beauty

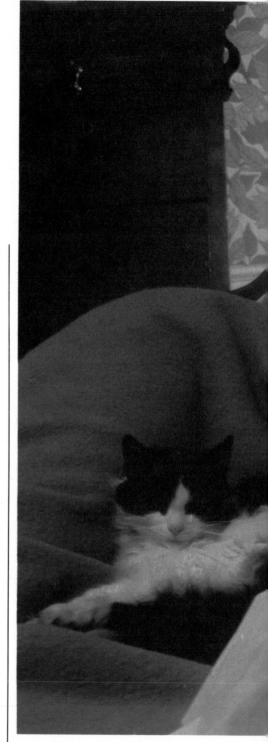

The body is a highly complex piece of machinery, and an efficient one too, if given the right kind of care. This must include the right diet and the correct amount of exercise and of sleep. A body which has all these things stands a strong chance of looking good and working well. If any one aspect is neglected, the body will respond by working inefficiently and the results of that may include dull hair, tiredness, irritability, splitting nails and other minor health problems. Although these may be only minor problems from a health point of view, they are major beauty problems. You will look attractive if you help your body to work well. And to do this, you need to understand one or two main points in beauty biology.

Sleep

Sleep helps us to restore our energy, to make the most of physical resources, to refresh our brains. The metabolic rate (the speed at which the body produces energy) slows down as we sleep, and the body exists with the minimum of activity. The amount of sleep necessary for each individual varies. Some people can awake refreshed from a comparatively short sleep — say, 4-6 hours. Others need much longer — as much as 10 hours. For growing children, the amount of sleep required is great, since the body has so much work to do while growth takes place.

Dreaming This, too, is a vital 'escape mechanism' for the body. It is now recognized that dreams help to release mental tensions and are an important aid to good health, especially in this high-pressure age. So, have plenty of sleep. You need it for health and beauty. Use it as the cheapest, simplest beauty treatment of all. Work out just how much you need for maximum benefit. If there are times when you have too little sleep, make sure that you replace the valuable hours lost during the next night. Try to space out late nights so that you can catch up on sleep in the interval. A series of very late nights, one after the other, takes a lot of your energy and is hard to recover from.

Your bed The way you prepare for sleep is important, too. Make sure your bed is comfortable. It should not be too soft: that is bad for your spine and not so comfortable as a firm mattress. Avoid mounds of pillows which could hasten the arrival of a double chin. If you can sleep without a pillow, or with just a single, flattish one, so much the better. Choose light yet warm bedclothes — a cellular blanket or a duvet [continental quilt] is better insulation than a pile of blankets and less constricting. Air the bed daily and use cotton sheets for cool comfort.

Preparing for sleep Before going to bed have a warm bath or a warm drink (or both) to encourage a relaxed sleepiness. Stretch out and lie fairly straight in bed. A hunched sleeping position can be bad for circulation and posture: we do after all spend a third of our lives in bed.

The kidneys

The kidneys are the 'clearing house' for the body's waste products. They lie high up on the back wall of the abdominal cavity, one on each side of the backbone. Their three main functions are important beauty treatments in themselves, as well as being essential to life:

1 The kidneys help to remove waste substances from the blood and excrete them from the body as urine. Cells in the body are continually breaking down, and new ones are being formed. Skin, for example, is constantly renewed, hair grows and so do nails. The waste substances from the breakdown of cells must be removed as soon as possible; otherwise the system would be poisoned. So they are carried by the blood to the kidneys to be filtered. Sugar, some salts and water are allowed to seep back into the blood and the waste products, together with some water, are formed into urine which passes to the bladder.

2 The kidneys help to regulate the amount of mineral salts in the blood. Even if our diet is perfectly balanced, we cannot entirely control the amount of any one mineral absorbed into the body. Our kidneys regulate this for us. As blood filters into the cup-shaped centres of the kidneys, its mineral content is regulated. If there is too much of a certain substance the kidneys

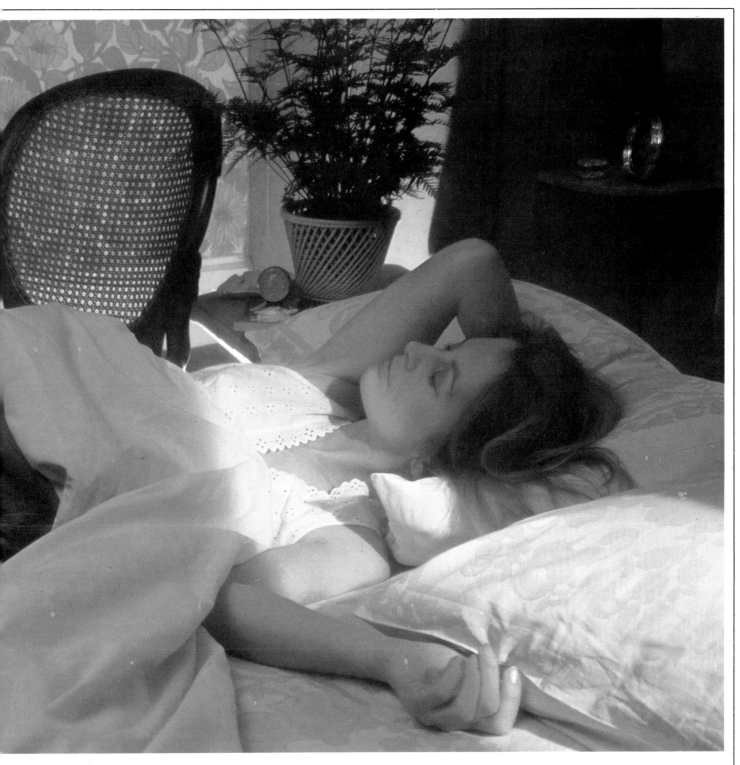

will retain it; if there is too little, they will replace the deficiency. However, the kidneys can only work with the material available. If someone is lacking in iron, for example, the kidneys cannot create this vital mineral. Many women are, in fact, iron-deficient during the child-bearing years (due to menstruation and child birth itself). Anaemia is the most obvious sympton of iron deficiency, but lesser symptoms connected with beauty like lethargy or dull hair and skin are very common.

3 The kidneys help to control the water balance of the body. There must be a precise balance between fluid taken into the body, and fluid lost as perspiration, as urine or as water vapour from the lungs. When the kidneys regulate the flow of fluid from the body as urine, they are following messages sent from the brain via a hormone produced by the pituitary gland. If too much fluid is present in the body, then a message is sent from the brain to the pituitary gland which produces a hormone carried by the blood to the kidneys. This hormone is a warning to the kidneys to increase the rate at which water is being excreted in the urine. If the body starts to

Sleep is the simplest, and one of the most effective, beauty treatments. Catch up on lost sleep quickly

lose too much fluid — by perspiring, for instance — the flow of hormone slackens, and the kidneys respond by excreting less water.

To keep the kidneys working well, drink about 1½ litres (3 pints) of fluid a day, and make sure that a good deal of that is plain water. If possible, try to drink some mineral water instead of tea and coffee. Both contain substances which the kidneys must filter out, and that gives them more to do.

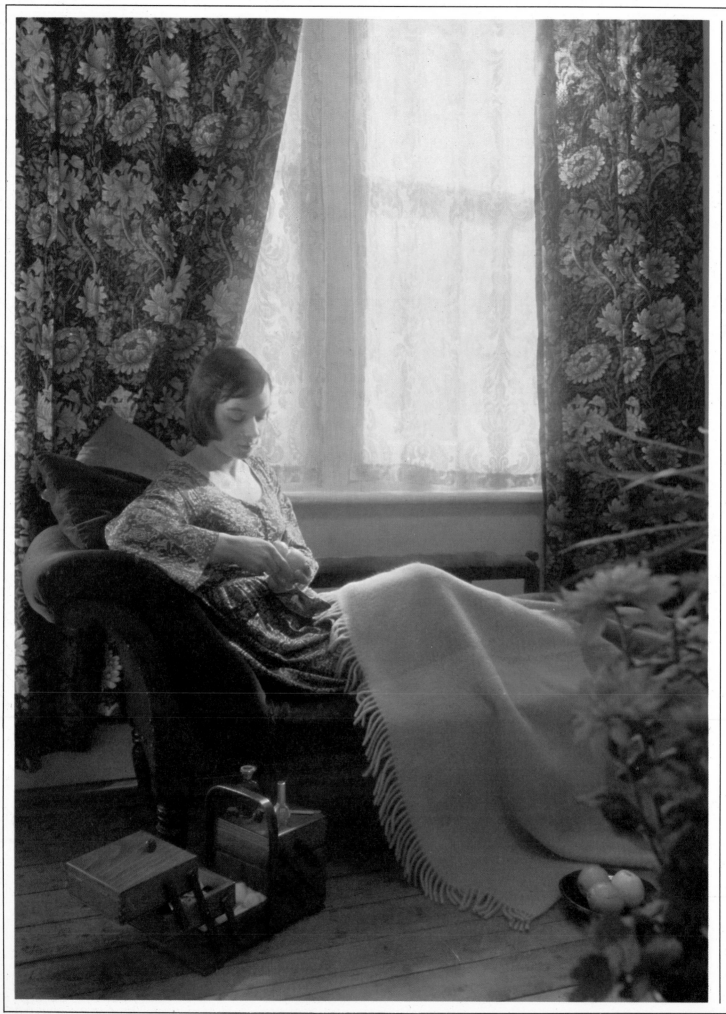

looking better than you feel

When we are not well, we are conscious of looking really unlovely — a very depressing feeling. When you have a bad cold, feel run-down, or are confined to bed with 'flu, it is still a good idea to keep to a beauty care routine, although the kind of cosmetics you use will be a little different from your usual ones, of course. There are make-up disguises and remedies which will improve your looks and consequently make you feel better much more quickly.

Colds and flu

Problems: red nose, cracked lips, dull hair and blotchy skin. Eyes often run too, making normal eye make-up impractical.

Solutions: If the cold is annoying, but hardly bad enough to keep you in bed, make a special effort to look good. Disguise blotchse and red nose with a green-tinged fonudation or powder worn over a moisturizer.

Soften lips with lip-balm and apply a very greasy, hypo-allergenic unperfumed lipstick while you have the cold. You will find that it needs re-applying quite often, but the effect is worth the effort. The lipstick should have a brownish tinge — not be too red or blue.

If your eyes look bleary and bloodshot, use an eye lotion or drops recommended by your doctor and a hypoallergenic waterproof mascara, lightly applied. Use a little powder eye shadow, but avoid colours like mauve, pink or blue. The best choices are browns, greys or soft greens.

Hair is usually a problem when you have a cold. If you do not feel like washing it, use a dry shampoo or a mixture of fuller's earth and talc brushed through your hair every few days until you feel well again. Brush the shampoo out of your hair very thoroughly, and put in a few rollers while you have a bath. When you see bounce in your hair you will feel much better.

If you are confined to bed, use the

When you feel below par, a regular beauty routine is a great morale-booster

dry shampoo routine to refresh your hair. Keep some eau-de-cologne or cologne-impregnated pads by your bedside. Freshen your face with a splash of skin tonic, apply moisturizer and a little green-tinged powder to disguise a red nose. If your cheeks look pale rub in a little peach-coloured blushing gel. Keep lips soft with lip balm and a little lip-gloss.

Try using waterproof mascara, even if you do not want the full eye make-up you usually wear. Give some thought to your nightdress or pyjamas — choose a cheerful colour. Keep a big bottle of mineral water or diluted unsweetened fruit juice by your bedside, too, to freshen your parched throat.

Post-natal care

Problems: Having a baby takes a great deal of energy. Even if you have been following a good ante-natal beauty programme you are bound to feel tired for the first few months after the birth of your child. Your skin may be dull and your hair lacking in shine.

Solutions: Be very careful to make sure that your diet is packed with nutrients: plenty of Vitamin C, protein and minerals. Keep up the iron supplement you took before your baby was born.

If your skin looks pale and sallow, use a pink-tinged make-up for a month or so to give you colour and add a little blusher. Take time from your new chores to put on eye make-up and lipstick every day: choose bright, pretty colours to cheer yourself up.

Your hair will need special care. Have it trimmed regularly and wash it frequently, using a conditioner at each shampoo. Try a semi-permanent tint in a colour near your own to add shine and body.

Watch your nails for cracking and splitting. Tackle all tough chores wearing rubber gloves. If your teeth are painful or dull-looking, see your dentist for a check up or a scale and polish treatment. Be lavish with perfume: if you have hoarded Christmas and birthday presents, now is the time to use them. And, finally, treat yourself

to at least one new outfit — as frivolous as you like.

Convalescence

Problems: Boredom, dull or sallow complexion, lifeless hair

Solutions: If you feel reasonably well, but are confined to bed to convalesce, use the time profitably to step up beauty care. Have a box of skin-care items in your bedside table, and pay special attention to cleansing and toning your skin each night. Put on a full make-up every morning, keeping it light with soft colours and skin-tones. Your nails will benefit particularly from this bedbound period, so make the most of them by giving them a complete manicure each week. Get someone to arrange all the things you need on a tray: polish, remover, orange sticks, nail file or emery boards, cuticle remover. Spread an old towel on the bed under the tray in case of accidents. Choose a pearl polish in a pinky shade. Ask a friend to help you wash and set your hair, too: shining hair will make you feel much better.

Rapid beauty boosters

Even if you're not actually ill, there may be times when you feel too tired and faded to care about your looks. Try one of these encouragements:

1 A dab of your favourite perfume at temples, wrists, behind your knees
2 A face-spray of mineral water (put some in an old perfume atomizer)
3 A long, relaxing bath scented with herbs
4 A professional pedicure
5 Ten minutes of yoga exercises
6 A short nap, with your feet resting on a pillow above the level of your head
7 A delicious beauty cocktail: 1 carton unsweetened yogurt, whisked with 3 tablespoons unsweetened blackcurrant juice, 1 spoonful of honey and a sprinkling of wheatgerm
8 A spur-of-the-moment visit to the hairdresser and a new hair-style
9 A 10-minute walk, followed by a warm bath
10 An appointment for a top-to-toe beauty treatment

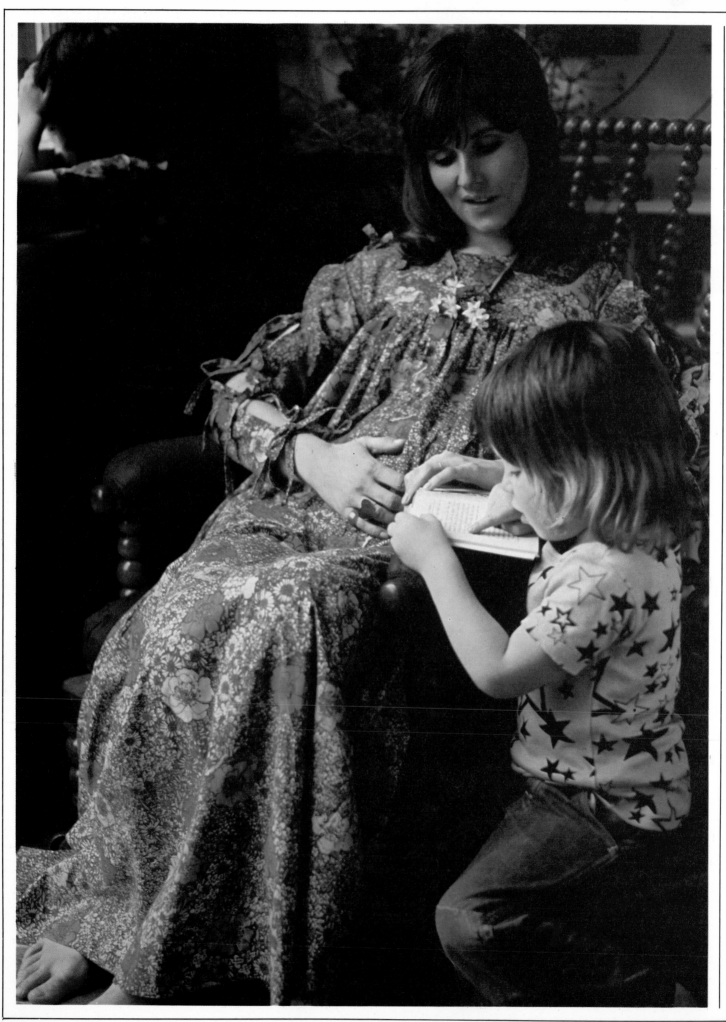

beauty while you wait

A woman can have a radiant serenity when she is pregnant. But pregnancy can also be a time of difficulty for a mother-to-be. There are additional physical strains to cope with and there can be mental ones, too. Adjustment to a different way of life can be a difficult process. Expenses may seem to increase alarmingly. Well-meaning friends and relatives may give confusing and often conflicting advice. In the midst of these pressures, is there room for beauty?

It is very important for an expectant mother to spend some of her time thinking about herself. If she is relaxed and healthy, then her baby stands a good chance of being healthy, too. The forty weeks of pregnancy have special beauty problems as well as some beauty bonuses. Nature is often very good at giving 'consolation prizes' so some mothers may find that pregnancy produces unexpected benefits like clear skin, or glowing cheeks and glossy hair. A expectant mother can make her pregnancy a rewarding and interesting experience from the beauty point of view, if she starts taking extra beauty care from the very beginning.

The first three months

This is the most difficult time for many mothers. Nausea, bad skin, lank hair — they all seem to happen at once. Now there is great hormonal activity in the body, which aggravates acne, lifeless hair and lack of energy.

In addition the figure becomes plump and lumpy: large enough to be too big to fit into ordinary clothes, but not yet big enough to need loose maternity clothes. The joy of realizing that you are pregnant may be clouded by doubts and disappointment over the way you look. Start by thinking positively about beauty care and by sticking to a strict daily beauty routine, which will help you to adjust to your new role and have a tremendous effect upon your looks and morale.

Skin-care If spots appear on your face, chest or back, don't worry. The increased hormonal activity in your body is causing this temporary upset. Clean skin thoroughly night and morning and treat spotty areas with astringent and a medicated skin lotion. Disguise the ones on your face with a medicated camouflage stick and apply a light make-up. Never squeeze any spot anywhere to get rid of it.

As soon as you know that you are pregnant, pay special attention to lubricating the skin on your stomach, buttocks and breasts. Apply plenty of skin conditioning cream after your bath and rub in baby oil or olive oil every night. Stretch marks are very difficult to remove after the birth, but lubrication of the skin now can prevent them altogether. Keep lubricating throughout the nine-month period.

Diet Forget the 'eating for two' myth. You need more nutrients, not more calories. Cut out fried, sweet, stodgy and fatty foods. The exception to this is fatty fish: they supply Vitamins A and D which you need now. Drink a pint of milk every day. If you dislike milk, make up the calcium requirement by increasing your intake of cheese.

Sometimes, morning sickness can be avoided by eating a small piece of dry toast or a digestive biscuit on waking. You may find, too, that smaller meals taken more frequently during the day help to prevent sickness pangs. Pander to food 'cravings' only if they are nutritionally correct!

Very often you will find that savoury foods appeal strongly to you. Indulge in them, by all means, but be wary of sudden desires for sugary foods. You could, subconsciously, be using the 'craving' as an excuse for eating incorrectly.

Always start the day with a good breakfast — a boiled egg, a slice of toast and orange juice with a cup of tea or coffee, for instance. If you are working, make sure that at lunchtime you eat lunch; do not rush about shopping. Try to include liver or kidney in your diet at least once a week. Avoid alcohol: you probably will not want it anyway.

Most of all, take the advice of your doctor. If he gives you iron pills, take them. In pregnancy, the body makes 25 per cent more blood than usual, so iron is vital. And you must build up calcium stores by drinking milk (or eating cheese). Otherwise, the growing baby will draw on your calcium to build his teeth and bones. This could mean severe dental trouble for you during and after your pregnancy.

Exercise Get as much fresh air as you can and take a good walk daily. Avoid really strenuous exercise during the crucial first three months; later it will be quite safe to resume a relaxing sport like swimming.

Rest Start organizing your day so that you can go to bed early. By 10.00 p.m. you will probably find that you feel very tired. Do not try to burn the candle at both ends — it will show in your face and your temper. Make up for the occasional late night by going to bed extra early the next night. This is a pattern that you should continue throughout your pregnancy. The most radiant mother-to-be of all is the rested one.

Hair-care If hair becomes lank and difficult, treat it to a good conditioning treatment. Think about having it re-styled in an easy-to-care-for shape now. Later, you will find that it becomes physically tiring to wash, dry and set a complicated hair-style. It is better to concentrate on good condition and a simple shape. If your hair is tinted, you may find it easier to have it re-tinted to a colour near to its natural one. You simply will not feel like spending hours sitting in hair salons under hot dryers.

The middle months

Beauty care taken early in pregnancy now begins to pay dividends. Most mothers find that nausea stops being a serious problem by the fourth month, and hair and skin conditions improve dramatically at this stage. If you have watched your diet carefully, your 'bump' will be a manageable size, too!

Skin-care Cleanse and tone skin twice a day, and apply moisturizer under your make-up. If cheeks look too rosy, tone them down with a green-tinged face powder over matt beige foundation. Don't overdo the toning down, however: flushed cheeks are all part of the healthy glow. Keep make-up basically simple, but experiment with different coloured eye shadows to match your clothes. Eyes should be bright and shiny now, so emphasize them.

Continue with daily stomach, bottom and breast lubrication and pay special attention to skin freshness.

You will feel warmer, so underarm depilation and deodorizing are essential. Make bathtime relaxing and enjoyable and follow every bath with a light foot massage to soften the skin and stimulate circulation. Night cramps are often a problem during the second half of a pregnancy.

Diet Keep up the same basic diet as before and watch your weight-gain carefully. Total weight-gain during pregnancy should be about 22 pounds. If yours is already coming dangerously near that mark, adjust your diet accordingly. Toxaemia (blood poisoning) and high blood pressure are dangers for overweight mothers-to-be, and so are varicose veins.

Exercise Keep walking, with your doctor's approval. Wear comfortable shoes and walk slowly and carefully. It is particularly important to keep up exercise if you stop working full time. Sit and sew and knit by all means, but do that in the evenings.

Rest You are probably in the habit of going to bed early now, so continue to do that. The most comfortable position in bed is lying on your side with one leg slightly in front of the other, one hand under the pillow and the other by your side. That way, the weight is evenly distributed. Bed-socks may seem unglamorous, but they can help to prevent night cramps.

Hair-care Your hair has probably settled down now and looking better than ever. Make the most of it by washing and setting it carefully, brushing it gently every day and using hair ornaments like combs, slides and bandeaux.

The final month

It may seem a long, long time since your pregnancy began. This is the month for organization, for the final preparations to welcome the baby. But take very good care of yourself, too: you will need a lot of energy in the coming months.

Skin-care Dryness and blotchiness are sometimes problems at the end of a pregnancy. Take care to nourish your skin nightly; use a covering foundation during the day. If your face looks fat, use shading to disguise the chubbiness. Give your body the luxury of plenty of skin cream this month. If you intend to breastfeed your baby, keep your nipples soft with a special cream to help prevent cracking.

Diet Increase milk and high-protein foods like fish, eggs, meat. Keep your iron intake high, too. This is the month for good food — but absolutely no stodgy extras. Drink fresh orange juice instead of tea or coffee to keep up your Vitamin C quota. This vitamin cannot be stored by the body, so supplies must be replenished daily. A high Vitamin C intake helps protect you against infections like colds and influenza, which you can well do without this month. When labour begins, have a good meal. You

will need. all your strength later on and you may not get another meal for many hours.

Exercise Walking is still good for you, as long as your doctor approves. However, take things slowly with a rest at frequent intervals.

Rest Take a short nap in the afternoons if you can, especially if you are planning to go out or to entertain in the evening. If you find it difficult to get to sleep, try a warm milky drink last thing at night or relax in a warm bath just before bedtime. However, do not take a bath when you are alone at home in case you slip or get stuck!

Hair-care Have your hair trimmed and set this month. You will be far too busy next month to go to the hairdresser's. Sit down when you are styling your hair, and if you have long hair, get someone else to brush it for you if it tires you to do it yourself. Hair may become a little greasy this month, so freshen it between shampoos by putting a piece of cheese cloth or muslin over the bristles of your brush and pressing them through it. Soak the fabric in cologne. Now brush your hair. Much of the dirt and grease will be caught on the fabric, which you can then throw away. This is a good hair freshener to keep in mind after your baby is born.

Post-natal exercise routine

After your baby is born, some gentle exercises will help you regain your pre-pregnancy figure quickly. It is safe to start these the day after the birth if there have been no complications, but check with your doctor or midwife before commencing. Repeat each day's exercises the next day, until by Day Six, you have the complete programme. Start with 6 to 8 movements on each; gradually increase to 20. Keep up programme until your tummy is flat, your waist measurement back to normal and your body muscles toned and firm.

Day one (first day after the birth) 1) Lie on your back on the bed, with hands palms-down by your sides, knees bent and feet flat. Breathe in and out rhythmically and evenly. Feel tummy muscles contracting with each breath. 2) Lie on back with legs straight, lift left leg slightly and rotate foot left, then right. Repeat with right leg. Tighten and relax knee muscles.

Day two 1) Lie on back with knees bent, hands palms-down by your sides. Tighten up abdominal muscles and buttocks, pressing the natural hollow out of your back at the same time. (This

is called the 'Pelvic Tilt'). 2) Lie with hands palms-down by your sides, legs crossed at the ankles. Now contract pelvic floor muscles. Hold briefly, then relax.

Day three 1) Lie on back with hands on hips, feet slightly apart. Draw up left hip and push down right hip simultaneously. Repeat, drawing up left hip and pushing down right hip. 2) Lie on your back with knees bent. Now raise your head and left arm so your left hand touches your right knee. Repeat with right arm and left knee. 3) If your doctor says you may get up today, try this easy exercise to correct the strange new balance of your body: Stand with your back against a wall, heels about 2 inches away, and push the small of your back and shoulders against it. Pull in tummy, relax shoulders and stand 'tall'. Keep knees braced, tail tucked in, chin down and head up.

Day four 1) Lie on your back, hands palms-down by your sides. Raise right leg and swing it over to the left so your right foot touches the left side of the bed. Swing the leg back to the centre, then lower again. Repeat with left leg, swinging to the right side of the bed this time.

2) Kneel on all-fours with back and arms straight. Hump your back; hold briefly; hollow it. Look up as you hollow, downwards as you raise up.

Day five 1) Lie on your back with feet together. Raise yourself up on left hand, lean forward and stretch hand to touch left ankle. Hold briefly, lie down again, then repeat with left hand touching right ankle.

2) Stand back against a wall, feet 2″ away, hands hanging loosely by your sides. Lean forwards from waist, so that trunk and head hang down loosely. Now gradually straighten up, feeling each 'knob' of backbone touch the wall as you uncurl your body. Relax shoulders and take a few deep breaths.

Day six 1) Kneel on all fours with back, head and arms straight. Slowly raise your right knee to 'touch' your nose (if you can't make it comfortably, do not strain. Just go as far as you can). Stretch your right leg backwards and then return to starting position. Repeat with left leg.

2) Lie on your back, hands palms-down by your sides. Raise left knee towards your tummy, hold briefly, stretch left leg upwards, then lower slowly. Repeat with right knee and leg.

ages of beauty

With correct skin care and diet, there is no reason why a woman should not look just as attractive at forty or fifty as she did at twenty, provided that she changes her style to suit her age-group. The biggest mistake that many older women make is to assume that a lipstick shade or eyeshadow which suited them ten years ago will still be right now. Skin tone and texture, hair colour and features all change gradually but noticeably as time passes. If, at any time, you feel that your attitude to make-up has become fixed, a professional make-up lesson with an expert will give you new ideas and fresh inspiration. At thirty or at forty a consultation with a beauty expert would make a useful and instructive present from you to you.

Here are general guidelines for skin care and make-up priorities at various ages:

The teens A time for experiment. Skin care routines learned now will stand you in good stead for the whole of your beauty life. Your hair styling may change from week to week — and so it should. Mistakes will be made — and this is the time for them.

The twenties A time for confidence. You have the experience to know what is right for you among the current make-up preparations and fashionable hairstyles, and you also have the confidence to try them. Skin care towards the end of this decade is particularly important. It is the time when fine lines start to appear.

The thirties and onwards This is a time for warmth and boldness. A complete switch in hair colour and make-up can make you feel renewed. Your body is probably in as good a shape now as it was in your twenties and if it is not, diet and exercise can help. Your whole attitude to life becomes more relaxed. You may be entertaining and going out more and this gives you chances to wear beautiful evening clothes, needing warm, beautiful make-up to complement them. A period of your life to enjoy to the full.

The three ages of beauty. Top left: the teens are the time to try new colours, new beauty ideas. Top right: the twenties are for confidence. Below: softness and warmth after 30

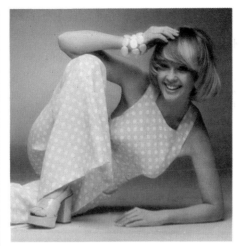

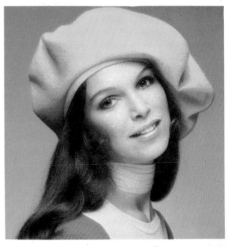

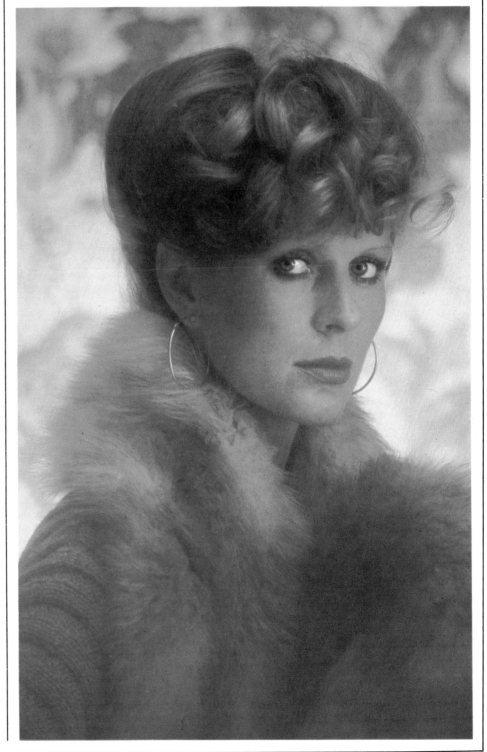

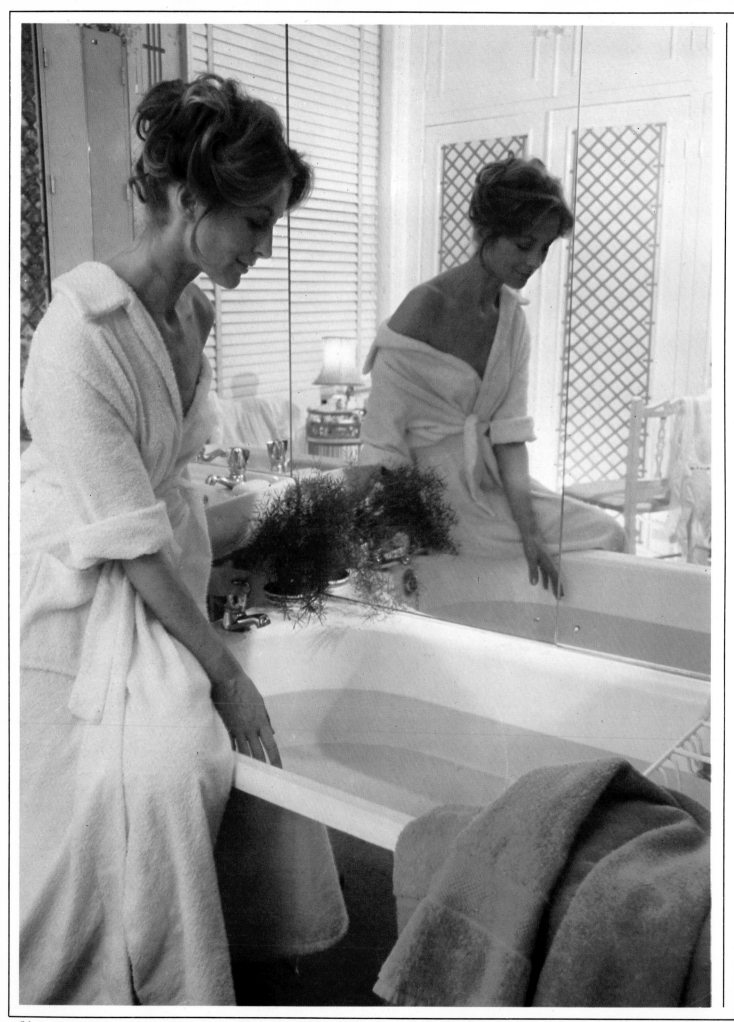

beauty and the bath

Every woman owes herself a little time each day to spend on her body. The easiest and least time-consuming way to achieve it is to combine your 'body beautiful' treatment with your bath. Choose a time at least once a week when you're likely to be undisturbed for 20 minutes or so and enjoy a real beauty treatment. Everything depends on a strict routine and the right equipment.

The twenty-minute luxury bath

Make sure that you have the following items:

Soft bath towel
Bath cap, bandeau or hair pins (to secure hair back from the face and off the shoulders and neck)
Bath robe and slippers
Friction mitt
Depilatory lotion or cream
Loofah or unscratchy bath brush
Bath oil or scented bubble bath
Soap and talc in a matching fragrance
Body lotion or massage cream
Pumice stone
Toenail clippers, orange sticks, cuticle cream
Anti-perspirant spray
Scented body cologne

Gather all these items together on a little table or a bathroom stool. Pour a little scented bath oil or bubble bath into the bath, and run the water. Don't make it too hot — 75°-80°F is hot enough. While the bath is running, undress, put on a bathrobe and tuck your hair away from your face and off your neck. Remove face make-up with cleansing lotion.

Take off your bathrobe, get into the bath and relax completely for a few minutes. Now soap the upper part of your body. Rub every part of it except your breasts with the friction mitt, paying particular attention to your neck. This usually neglected area sometimes becomes grey-looking because of bad circulation. Rubbing with the mitt will help to improve this. Give care to your upper arms, elbows and shoulders, too. Now use the loofah to give your back a thorough scrub, and help to prevent spots. Use the friction mitt again on legs, bottom, heels and ankles. Relax again completely for at least five minutes before stepping out of

the bath. Towel your body dry by patting and rubbing it very gently, and apply scented talc under arms, on feet and on the pubic area. With firm, gentle strokes, rub body lotion or massage cream into the rest of your body. Use both hands to rub it in well over back, bottom, breasts, stomach, legs and arms. Put on your bathrobe. Lay several tissues on a towel on the bathroom stool. Place one foot on the tissue and examine for hard skin. Rub away gently and firmly with pumice, then trim toenails with clippers (the clippings can be wrapped up in the tissues afterwards).

Ease back cuticles with an orange stick and cuticle cream. Repeat the process for the other foot, then rub in plenty of body lotion.

If depilation (de-fuzzing) of your legs or underarms is unnecessary, use an anti-perspirant spray now, followed by a liberal splashing of perfumed cologne all over your body. If depilation is necessary, apply the cream now, relax for a few minutes, then wash it off.

Do not apply anti-perspirant before or immediately after depilation: dust a little more talc under your arms instead and use the anti-perspirant later in the day. On legs, a moisturizing cream is particularly necessary after depilation, as the skin tends to be dry. Rub in plenty of lotion with firm, upward strokes.

After your bath, try to relax on your bed for a few minutes before making-up and dressing again. After relaxing, if you have time to sit (in your bathrobe) and give yourself a manicure or pedicure or both before dressing, then do.

The ten-minute daily beauty bath

The morning is the best time for this. Gather together the items in the checklist for the twenty-minute beauty bath (leaving out the depilatory lotion, pumice stone, toenail clippers, orange sticks and cuticle cream). Have them ready with your dressing-gown, underclothes and tights.

Run your bath and add the bath oil or bubble bath. Then go back into your bedroom to take off your nightclothes, make your bed and lay out what you

are going to wear for the day. Pin curl hair and put on bathcap. Make sure that the bath water is not too warm. Step into the bath, soap your body all over, then run briskly with the friction mitt. Use the loofah on your back. Relax for just a few seconds. Step out quickly and rub yourself down briskly with the bath towel. Cool off for a moment. Apply talc to the pubic area and a little body lotion everywhere else. Use the anti-perspirant under your arms. While you're waiting for it to dry, clean your teeth and your face. Splash some refreshing cologne all over your body to make you feel tinglingly fresh. Put on your underclothes, tights (or stockings) and dressing gown. Then back to your bedroom to make up and put on the rest of your clothes.

Five-minute daily beauty shower

This is the quickest routine of all and very invigorating.

Have these items ready:
Underclothes and tights (or stockings)
Bath cap
Shower gel or soap
Soft bath towel
Dressing gown
Body lotion
Friction mitt
Loofah
Scented body cologne
Anti-perspirant spray
Talc

Take off your nightclothes in the bathroom, and pull on bath cap. Pin curl your hair first if you have time. Switch on the shower, making sure that it isn't too hot. Apply the shower gel, then step under the water. Rub your body down with the friction mitt, apart from your breasts, of course. Use the loofah on your back. Gradually adjust the shower so that it becomes cooler or even cold if you can stand it. The coolness will close your pores and help you to shake off a sluggish, early morning feeling.

Switch off the shower and step out. Rub your whole body down with the towel, then apply talc to the pubic area and body lotion everywhere else. Use the anti-perspirant under your arms. Clean your teeth and cleanse your face. Splash scented cologne all over.

be your own beautician

From time to time, when you have a whole day to yourself — a Sunday, perhaps, or an odd day of holiday — devote it to beauty. Even in such a short time, there are many beauty jobs that you can do and you will end the day looking and feeling totally relaxed and refreshed. Begin by making sure that you go to bed fairly early the night before your day of beauty. Have a warm bath and a hot drink to make you sleep soundly. Set the alarm clock for 8.30 a.m.

A day for beauty

8.30 a.m. Breakfast: Drink the juice of half a lemon in hot sugarless water.
8.45 a.m. Limbering exercises in front of an open window, followed by deep breathing. Then total relaxation on the floor for 1 minute.
9.00 a.m. Lukewarm shower or bath. Dress in jeans and a sweater or T-shirt and comfortable shoes. Apply moisturizer and a little eye make-up. No heavy foundation or powder today.
9.20 a.m. Light Breakfast: Unsweetened orange juice, 1 boiled egg, starch-reduced crispbread with a scraping of butter, coffee or tea with milk but no sugar.
10.00 a.m. The next two hours must be devoted to some form of exercise such as swimming, riding or walking. You need to go out in the fresh air, even if it's raining. Do not worry about what you look like: you will wash your hair and re-do your make-up in the afternoon.
12.00 noon Check that you have all the equipment you need for the afternoon: shampoo, de-fuzzing cream (if you use it), tweezers for plucking eyebrows, orange sticks, nail file, bath oil and lotion, a selection of make up. This should include all the items you have been meaning to try.
12.30 p.m. Light lunch: raw vegetable salad (grated carrot, shredded cabbage, cauliflower sprigs, chopped celery, watercress, cucumber) with lemon juice dressing, 1 carton of cottage cheese. A fresh orange to follow. Tea or coffee (with milk but no sugar).
1.15 p.m. Rest for three quarters of an hour, with your feet slightly higher than your head, on your bed.
2.00 p.m. Change into a housecoat and prepare to make your bedroom and

bathroom your headquarters for the next three hours. Remove make-up with a cleanser. Take a medium-sized mixing bowl into the bathroom. Stand it on a table and almost fill it with very hot water. Lean your face close to the bowl, having first draped a towel over your head so that it and the bowl are enclosed in a kind of towelling tent. Stay under the towel so that your face has a sauna treatment for some minutes, while the steam from the bowl remains hot. Afterwards relax for a few minutes to allow your face to cool. Splash with a mild astringent. Apply a face pack that suits your skin type. Relax for ten minutes.
2.30 p.m. Remove face pack with tepid water. Splash face with astringent again. Apply moisturizer or special treatment cream if your skin is exceptionally dry. Run your bath, pouring in plenty of bath oil or bubble bath.
3.00 p.m. Relax in the bath. Rub your body (apart from your bosom) with a friction mitt to stimulate circulation. Relax. Your skin will get the full benefit of the moisturizer or treatment cream which will penetrate deep into the pores. After your bath, de-fuzz legs and underarms. Give yourself a full-scale pedicure. Put on housecoat, underclothes and tights again.
3.45 p.m. Devote the next hour to make-up experiments. Match the colour of your clothes with the new cosmetics. Look at the clothes you will wear in the next few days and see if any need cleaning or washing. Pluck your eyebrows, following the instructions in Making Beautiful Eyes. Keep the balance of your face in mind as you do it.
4.45 p.m. Cleanse your face thoroughly once more. Collect the equipment you need to wash and set your hair. Try a conditioner if you have dry, fly-away hair or a lemon rinse for greasy hair. Set your hair.
5.15 p.m. Dry hair using a hood or hair-dryer on a stand so that your hands are free. While your hair dries give yourself a complete manicure.
6.00 p.m. After completing the manicure, make up your face — lightly if you plan to spend the evening at home, more thoroughly you are going out. Brush out your hair carefully.
6.45 p.m. Dress in a caftan or housegown if you are staying at home. Put on your favourite evening clothes if

you are going out.
7.30 p.m. A light meal at home: Fruit juice or half a grapefruit (without sugar), fish, steak or chops with two green vegetables; a piece of fresh fruit or a fresh fruit salad. Tea or coffee (with milk but no sugar).
8.30 p.m. Relax with a magazine or book (no television this evening).
10.00 p.m. Go to bed. (This may happen a little later if you have been out for the evening.)

Two days for beauty

In two days, a great deal of beauty care can be achieved. If possible ask a friend to join you: the weekend will be more enjoyable if you can compare notes and progress with someone else.

In the preceding week

Quite early in the week, book a session at your local beauty or health club for a sauna and massage on Saturday afternoon. These treatments are becoming very popular, so it is wise to book in advance.

Friday evening

Try to organize all your weekend chores tonight, so that you have Saturday and Sunday completely free. Make sure you have the following items: a swimsuit, jeans, sweater and comfortable shoes, shampoo and conditioner; bath oil; talc; leotard for exercising. Add the following items to your Friday shopping list: 8 oranges; 1 large bottle of mineral water; 2 lemons; 1 large carton of cottage cheese; some fresh fruit.
Relax during Friday evening. Try to be in bed by 10.00 p.m.

Saturday

8.0 a.m. On waking, stretch thoroughly in bed. Get up and spend five minutes on exercises, concentrating on your 'problem' areas (see Areas for Special Care). Have a shower, or a quick bath. Dress in jeans (or slacks) and sweater.
8.30 a.m. 2 oranges, 1 glass of mineral water. Eat the oranges slowly and sip the water slowly, too.
9.00 a.m. Do any necessary shopping.

Go home to get swim suit.

10.00 a.m. Enjoy an hour at your local swimming pool. The breast stroke is good for bust, arms, stomach and thighs; the back stroke strengthens shoulder and leg muscles. Be vigorous in your swimming: don't merely float about lazily.

11.30 a.m. Early Lunch: Cottage cheese and a salad of mixed fruit and vegetables with lemon juice dressing. Sip mineral water after your meal.

1 p.m. Rest for half an hour with your feet higher than your head.

1.30 p.m. Take a brisk walk, wearing warm clothes if the weather is cold.

3.30 p.m. Keep the sauna and massage appointment. Relax totally during the afternoon.

5.30 p.m. Snack: 1 carton yogurt (natural and unsweetened), 1 orange and some mineral water. Allow yourself one cup of tea (unsweetened) if you must.

6.30 p.m. Wash and set your hair very carefully (using the methods described in the sections on Hair).

8.00 p.m. Put on a casual caftan or house gown. Apply a light make-up and spend the evening relaxing.

9.00 p.m. Eat another orange and sip more mineral water.

10.00 p.m. Cleanse face thoroughly. Use two applications of lotion. Tone and nourish to suit your skin type.

Sunday

8.30 a.m. On waking, stretch thoroughly in bed. Spend five minutes on the special 'problem area' exercises. Take a lukewarm bath or shower. Dress in underclothes and housecoat.
Breakfast as Saturday.

10.00 a.m. Sunday morning is to be devoted to your face. Give yourself a facial sauna (see A Day for Beauty — 2.00 p.m.) Relax for a few minutes. Pluck eyebrows very carefully and remove any chin hairs. Brush eyebrows into place with a small brush.
Experiment with new make-up techniques for half an hour, making sure that you work in a good light. Consider the clothes in your wardrobe while you work. Here a friend can be a great help by giving unbiased advice.
Tidy your make-up bag and/or drawer thoroughly. Discard any half-finished pots of shadow and creams which you won't be using again. Reorganize the equipment you have left and make a note of missing things.

1.00 p.m. Have lunch but avoid all starchy foods, and eat an extra helping of green vegetables. For dessert, have a large helping of fresh fruit salad. Finish with a glass of mineral water.

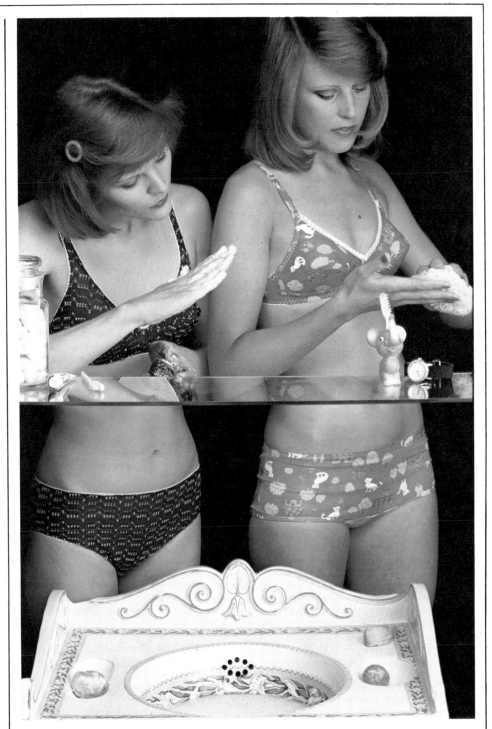

2.30 p.m. Put on jeans (or slacks) and sweater and take a long walk. Make sure that you have comfortable shoes. Watch your posture while you walk and breathe deeply and evenly.

4.30 p.m. Give yourself a complete manicure. Take ample time and apply three coats of polish, waiting at least 10 minutes between each coat.

5.30 p.m. A snack of 1 carton of natural yogurt, 1 orange and a glass of mineral water. Drink a cup of (unsweetened) tea, if you must.

6.30 p.m. Change into a leotard and spend half an hour on exercises.

7.00 p.m. Collect all you need for a beauty bath and pedicure. (See the Keeping Fresh and Pedicure sections.)

It's fun to plan a beauty weekend with a friend. Share make-up ideas, eat healthy foods together, encourage each other to exercise. A little rivalry helps too!

8.30 p.m. Put on a caftan or house gown, brush your hair and apply perfume and a light make-up. Relax. During the evening eat one orange and sip a glass of mineral water.

10.00 p.m. Go to bed.
After these two days, your scales should register a weight loss of up to 4 pounds. Your skin will look good and your hair, finger nails and toe nails will all be well-groomed. You will feel — and look — better and consequently more beautiful.

cosmetic surgery

A very obvious physical defect, such as an ugly nose, a drooping bosom or deep bags under the eyes, can undermine self-confidence and so spoil the pleasure of life generally. If it causes constant anxiety, there is good sense in considering cosmetic surgery.

Often the defect may look less embarrassing than it feels but the surgery may still be worthwhile simply to rebuild confidence. Surgeons are becoming more and more skilful in remoulding faces and figures, but anyone contemplating a surgical operation should be warned that the time involved can be lengthy and the treatment itself costly. A nose reshaping, for instance, would probably cost as much as a luxury holiday.

Eye bags

Double or triple bags under the eyes give an aging impression which is very unflattering. A skilled surgeon can smooth the skin with a single 'tuck' at the outer corner of the eye which hardly shows. This operation usually means an overnight or two-day stay in a hospital or clinic. The eyes are bandaged for about 24 hours, and when the bandages are removed the skin beneath the eyes will look pinkish for a few days. It is unadvisable to use make-up on the area or touch it for several weeks, until the tiny scars are completely healed.

Bosom

If your bosom is too small, its shape and size can be improved with the insertion of small silicone-packed bags under the skin. The operation is only done after careful consultation and demands a two- or three-day stay in hospital. Small scars on the lower part

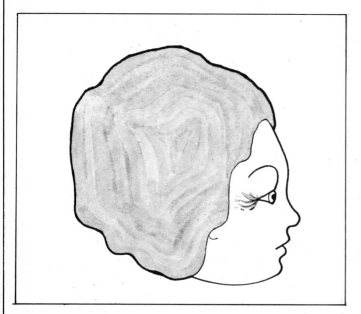

Above: *Wrinkles at the corners of the eyes are called 'laughter lines' or 'crow's feet'*

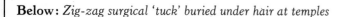
Below: *Zig-zag surgical 'tuck' buried under hair at temples*

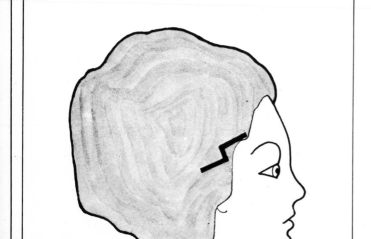

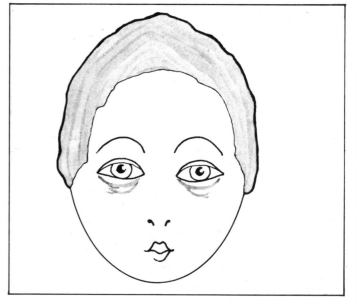

Above: *'Bags' below the eyes are one of the most telling signs of aging*

Below: *Surgical 'tuck' taken just below the lower eyelashes*

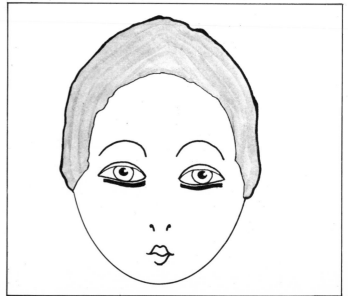

of the bust, towards the outer edge usually, are the only evidence of the operation. However, after the operation, the breasts need regular medical check-ups to make sure that all is well beneath the skin's surface.

If the bosom is too droopy, a tuck can be taken in the skin-fold above each breast, and slack skin removed. The post-operative care must again be thorough and no strain put on this whole area of the body for several weeks.

Face

Slack, wrinkled skin on the face can be smoothed out with a face lift. Two sets of 'tucks' are usually needed: one behind each ear and one at each temple (often set back in the hairline where they are easily concealed).

A three- or four-day stay in a hospital or clinic is necessary for the actual operation. Then, until the scars have healed—three or four weeks at the minimum—there must be great care. Although this operation can be repeated several times quite safely, the pulling action to create the tucks may make the eyes look slit-like in time.

Nose

This is one of the commonest operations since so many people are dissatisfied or embarrassed by the size or shape of their nose. The surgeon will usually give a preliminary consultation and will photograph your nose. However, no responsible surgeon will be able to give you more than a brief idea of just how your altered nose is going to look: so much depends on what is discovered on the operating table. The nose bone has to be broken, then reset, and although the stay in hospital may be only four or five days, it could be several months before the swelling has totally subsided. After the operation the nose is bandaged and the rest of the face may be heavily bruised. The speed of recovery and healing depends on the individual: usually, the younger you are the more quickly you recover. There may, however, be post-operative depression and for a few days breathing may be affected.

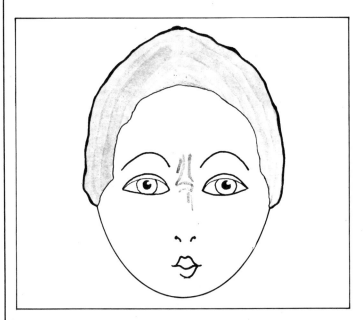

Above: *'Concentration' wrinkles between the eyes*

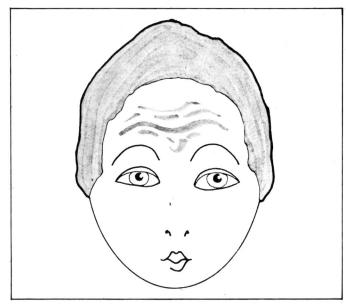

Above: *Frown lines on the forehead before surgery*

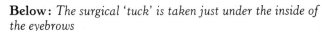

Below: *The surgical 'tuck' is taken just under the inside of the eyebrows*

Below: *Incision is made from temple to temple under eyebrows and surgical 'tuck' taken just inside the hairline*

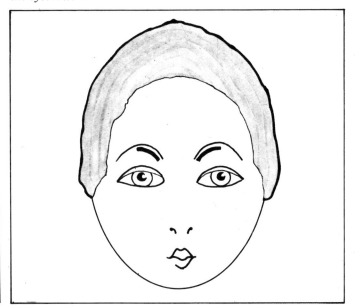

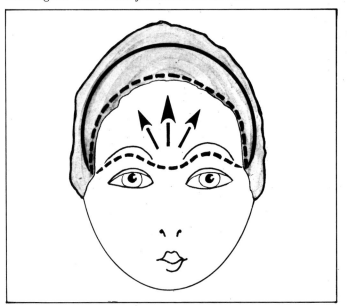

the perfume for you

The traditional home of the perfume industry is in France, in the Provence town of Grasse. Here the precious oils and essences are collected, distilled and blended. Most manufacturers, when they are considering the introduction of a new perfume, will turn first to the experts in Grasse for a perfect new blend which expresses exactly the effect they want.

Perfumes are generally costly because the preparation of the essences for them is a long and complicated process.

Many of the flower ingredients — jasmine, for example — are expensive to grow and have to be gathered at dawn when their fragrance is at its strongest.

Making certain that the fragrance stays in the perfume is a complex matter, too, requiring the use of what are called fixatives. In the past, the fixative used was civet, a glandular substance secreted by the civet cat, found mainly in Ethiopia. This is now a rare animal, so synthetic fixatives have to be manufactured and used. Musk is another costly ingredient. Natural musk has to be collected from the sex organs of the female musk deer. Now that much importance is attached to the preservation of wild animals, only a very few perfumes still contain natural musk, and its costliness makes it a rarity, too.

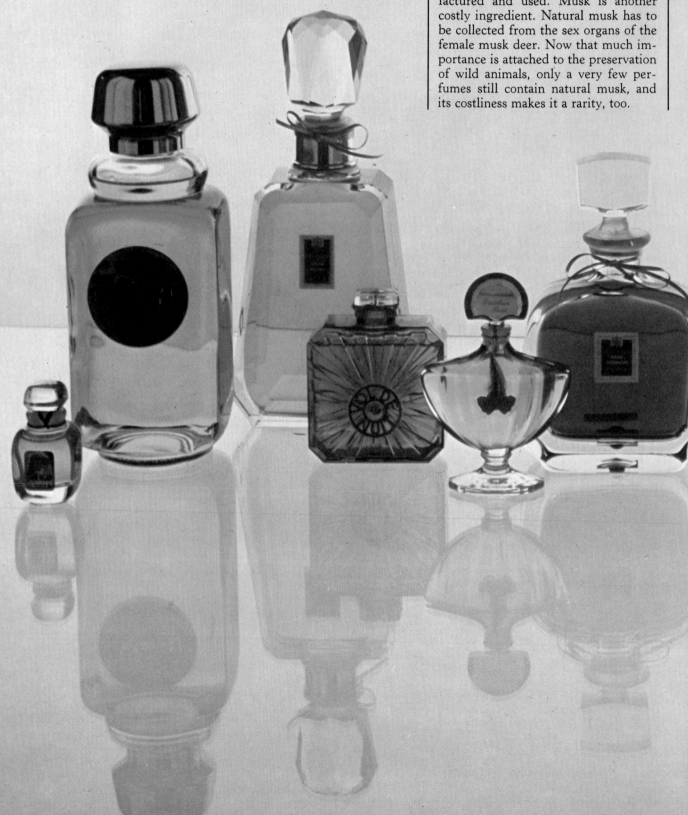

Because it is often literally so precious, perfume should be treated and used with care. Keep it in a place without strong light: direct sunlight will cause it to evaporate. Use it up: making it last by leaving it in its flask is not a real economy, since its characteristic fragrance will become muted and flat in time.

In the daytime, make liberal use of a cologne which matches your perfume. Heighten the fragrance by putting some of the actual perfume on your throat, on your wrists and behind your ears. In the evening, if you are entertaining or going out, put on more perfume in these same places, to add depth and richness to the fragrance.

If you are undecided about how to choose a perfume to express your individuality, or if you want to make a change in the fragrance you usually use, consult the perfume chart here for help.

A quick guide to choosing — or changing — your perfume. After each of the three broad groups of characteristics below, there is a list of some of the fragrances that suit them.

Gaiety: A quick, changeable mind: Enthusiasm: A liking for what is new: Sociability: A pleasure in sport: Vitality: Self-confidence

Musk: Amber: Spice: Patchouli: Jasmine: Rose: Carnation: Orchid

Gentleness: A liking for soft colours: Artistic ability: Home-loving: A romantic sense of the past: A subtle gift for organization: A quiet manner: Feminity
Jonquil: Honeysuckle: Gardenia Lavender: Violet: Lilac: Narcissus: Geranium

Sophistication: Ability to organize: Energy: A pleasure in outdoor life: Orderliness: Realistic self-knowledge: A taste for success: Good sense Lemon: Orange blossom: Lily of the valley: Musk: Sandalwood: Tuberose: Attar of roses: Carnation

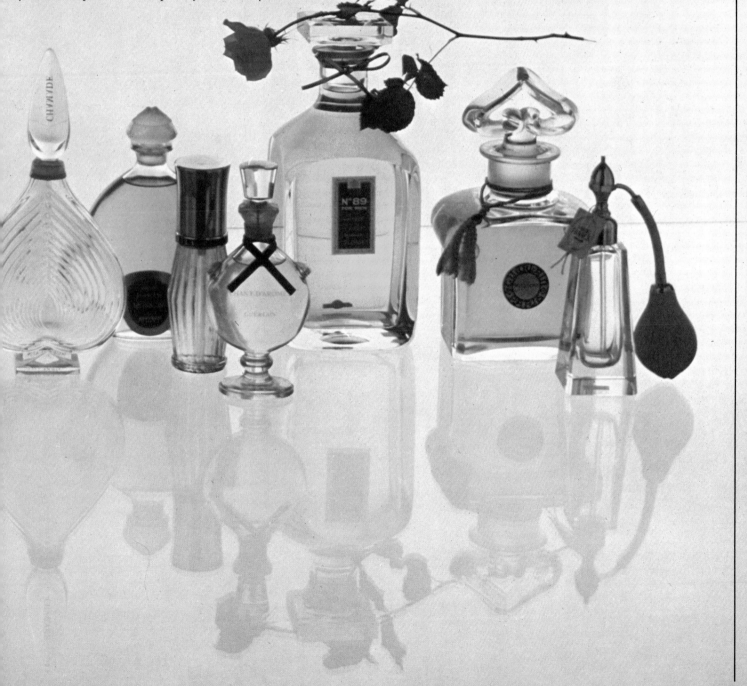

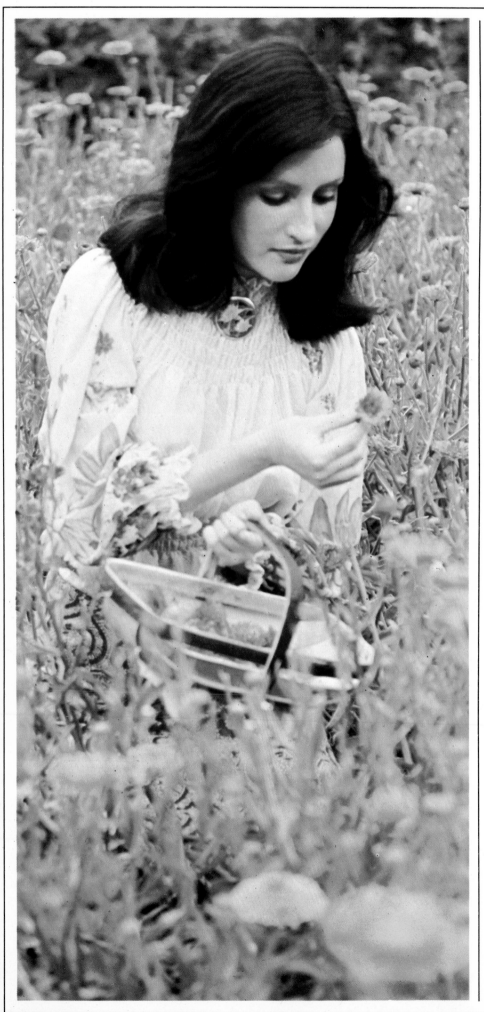

food for beauty

Today the range of cosmetics is tremendous. In the past, women needed to make good use of all kinds of everyday items — fruits, vegetables, nuts, cereals — in caring for their beauty. Here is an alphabetical list of fascinating recipes for you to try.

Apples

Best as a toner for oily skin. Use as a face mask: grate a large apple very finely and spread a layer all over your face, preferably when you are lying down. Leave on for 15 minutes, then wash off.

Almonds

Almond oil is good for both dry hair and dry skin. (Ground almonds or almond meal can be used in face masks.)
Large Pores Mix a tablespoonful of almond meal with enough water to make it easy to spread, and rub into the skin, like beauty washing grains. Leave it on as a mask for 15 minutes. Rinse off with tepid water.
Dry hair Warm two tablespoons of almond oil in a cup, standing in a pan of hot (not boiling) water. Massage the oil into hair, cover the scalp with a plastic bag, then with a hot damp towel and leave in place for 30 minutes. Remove oil with a mild shampoo.
Violet cold cream (the ingredients come from your larder and a chemist) 1 oz white wax, 5 fl oz sweet almond oil, 1 oz spermaceti, $1\frac{1}{2}$ fl oz rose water, 10 grains borax, $\frac{1}{2}$ teaspoon essence of violets.
Grate the wax and spermaceti finely and melt together, heating gently. Add the almond oil. Remove the heated ingredients from the stove and pour in rose water, in which you have already dissolved the borax. Beat mixture briskly and when it begins to thicken, add the violet essence. Put in a large jar with a screw top before the mixture cools.
Soften dry skin on both hands and face, with 1 oz of ground almonds. Add a cup of cold milk to the almond, a little at a time. Stir thoroughly, then strain (through muslin). Add $\frac{1}{2}$ oz sugar. Use the mixture to smooth on

Marigolds have long been used to make a refreshing and healing skin tonic face and hands. Leave on for 15 minutes. Wash off with tepid water.

Avocado

Avocado is rich in oil. Mexican women use it to protect their skins, it is an ingredient in creams and cosmetics, and you can use the fruit to soothe and smooth dry skin. Eat the avocado flesh first, then rub the skins over face (keeping them away from the eyes in case of smarting) and any part of the body that seems dry.

Avocado face mask Mash a ripe avocado with 1 teaspoonful of lemon juice and the white of an egg until soft enough to apply. Leave on the face for 20 minutes. Wash off with tepid water.

Barley

The powdered variety of barley can be mixed with 2 teaspoonsful of lemon juice and a little milk to make a face mask. This will improve the circulation and give a deep cleanse.

Age-old hand treatment: 1 oz honey, white of 1 egg, 1 teaspoonful of glycerine mixed with ground barley and rubbed in to the skin of hands.

Beer

A proved and favourite rinse to give your hair body and to make it manageable for setting (stale beer is best).

Bran

Sewn into a bag and used in the bath, bran was an old remedy for dry skin. Leave the bag to soak in your bath water for a while, then squeeze out the water absorbed by the bag, too.

For open pores Make a small bag out of a piece of flannel and put in about four tablespoons of bran and the shredded peel from two lemons. Put the bag into boiling water for a few seconds. Remove it. Dab your face with it.

Buttermilk

This has been a beautifier for almost as long as there have been cows! Milkmaids probably discovered its benefits and then passed on the good news. Mix a tablespoon or two of oatmeal with enough buttermilk to make a smooth consistency. Apply this to the face. Leave for 20 minutes. Rinse away.

Open pores Soak a cotton wool pad in buttermilk and pat on face. Leave the milk for about 10 minutes. Wash off with cold water.

To get rid of freckles Pat on buttermilk and leave to dry. (No one seems to know why this should work, but it has been a recommended beauty recipe for hundreds of years.)

Carrots

These are not only full of vitamins for inside health, but can be used as a beauty treatment, too. Dr Erno Laszlo, an Hungarian skin specialist who is well known in America for the use of natural food ingredients in his beauty preparations, suggests a carrot and turnip face mask. Cook the vegetables, mash and spread the cooled paste on the skin for 30 minutes. Wash off. (He has also suggested washing the face in a mixture of carrot and tomato juice.)

Castor oil

Much pleasanter for outside use! It can lubricate eyebrows and eyelashes, condition dry hair, aid dry skin, and help to strengthen nails. Fill an empty, clean nail varnish bottle with oil, add three or four drops of white iodine, shake well, and paint nails with the mixture twice a day.

Cocoa butter and coconut oil

The coconut oil makes a good hair conditioner. Used as a gentle body rub, it will help you to keep a tan. Cocoa butter is a splendid emollient, good for massaging in hands or face. Make Crème Simon, a nourishing skin cream, with 2 oz cocoa butter, 1½ fl oz elderflower water, 2½ fl oz rose water, 2 oz lanolin and 2 oz glycerine. Make your own cocoa butter cream with white wax, spermaceti, almond oil and cocoa butter.

Cosmetic (cider) vinegar

In Victorian times people soaked wraping paper in cider vinegar and applied it to their temples to keep the skin round the eyes smooth and free from wrinkles. Today some experts believe that cosmetic vinegar helps to protect the natural acid in the scalp and the skin. Every time you wash your face and body or shampoo your hair you wash away some of the natural acid which acts as a covering to protect you against infection.

Take 2 heaped tablespoons dried peppermint leaves. Put into 1 pint of water. Bring to boil and simmer for 2 minutes. Remove from heat. Strain, mix with 1 pint of cider vinegar. Leave for 48 hours before use. Put in the bath (half a cup) and in the final rinsing water after shampooing.

Cream

The kind of cream you eat can be mixed with mashed strawberries for a delicious and beautifying summer mask.

Cucumber

Naturally astringent and cooling, cucumber juice plays a large part in natural beauty treatments. It is used for toning, refreshing, for the treatment of big pores, and for cooling sunburn. Extract the juice by grating the cucumber finely, or liquidizing in an electric blender. Alternatively cut it up into small pieces, cover with hot water, simmer for half hour and strain.

Make a compress for the face by soaking gauze in the cold juice. Take 3 fl oz juice and mix with 2 fl oz distilled witch hazel and 1½ fl oz rose water to make a skin freshener. Dab an oily nose and chin with a pad of cotton wool soaked in cucumber juice.

Cucumber cold cream: 2 oz almond oil added to ½ oz shredded white wax. Dissolve in a fireproof bowl standing in a saucepan of boiling water. Peel and chop cucumber (about one quarter of a whole one). Add to the oil and wax mixture and simmer slowly for about an hour, covering the bowl. Stir and remove from heat. Cool and store in pots with screw top lids.

Eggs

Eggs are one of the oldest of beauty aids. The whites are toning and tightening, the yolks nourishing and enriching. An old recipe for a mask uses egg white mixed with 3 oz ground barley and 1 oz honey. A simple alternative: apply raw egg white to a clean skin. Leave to dry. Rinse off with luke warm water.

Put mayonnaise on your face and it will do it the world of good. This is especially true for dry skins. Make your own with 2 egg yolks, ½ cup sunflower oil, ½ cup sesame oil, 1 tablespoon wheat germ oil, 1 tablespoon herb vinegar, 2 drops of perfume or rose geranium oil. Use the mixture for cleansing, for smoothing dry patches, and for feeding the skin after sunbathing.

Another cleanser: the yolk of an egg mixed with 2 teaspoons of almond oil. Mix dried skimmed milk, egg white and a drop of camphor to make a tightener for the skin of the neck.

A hair conditioner Beat up two eggs in a wine glass of rum to produce a shine. Leave the mixture on your hair for 15 minutes. Rinse off with luke warm water.

Honey

An item used in many beauty treatments. It is excellent for smoothing the skin and softening lines.

You can spread it as a film all over the face. Leave on for 15 minutes and remove with cotton wool pads and warm water. Another use is to mix it with other ingredients to make face packs.

For dry skin A honey and egg mask: ½ teaspoon honey, 1 egg yolk, 1 tablespoon dry skimmed milk. Mix to a paste with a little fresh milk if necessary. Apply to the face and neck. Leave on for 15 minutes. Rinse off with tepid water.

For oily skin Mix ½ teaspoon honey with a dessertspoon lemon juice. Mix to a paste with fuller's earth or powdered barley, adding a little water if necessary to get the right spreading consistency.

Lemons

One of nature's most frequently used beauty additives, lemons have a bleaching, astringent action. They can be too drying for sensitive, parched skins, but very good for oily, blemished ones. Add milk and lemon juice to oatmeal to make a mask that will deep cleanse and liven your skin colour.

After a shampoo, put lemon juice in the final rinsing water to brighten blonde hair. Use a mixture of 1 teaspoon lemon juice and 2 tablespoons rose water to whiten grey elbows or to liven dingy skin.

Marigolds

One of the oldest aids to beauty.

For a skin tonic Make an infusion of marigold flowers: 1 oz of petals to 1 pint of water. Heat them together slowly (in an enamel or stainless steel pan). Keep the pan covered so that no steam escapes. Let the liquid cool for some hours. Strain it into a glass container with a screw-top. Use as a cleansing and healing lotion.

Melons

Melons have a cooling effect, wonderfully refreshing on a hot day. Slice off thin pieces and rub them over the face or put the slices between layers of gauze and use as a face compress—relaxing with the compress over your face for 15 minutes.

Milk

Half a pint of milk, mixed with the juice of 1 lemon can be used as a face lotion at night.

An old recipe for soothing sunburn was to pat the skin with a lotion made from ¼ pint of milk, into which had been added a pinch of bicarbonate of soda.

For dry skin A milk and honey mask, mixed with ground almonds.

For oily skin A face pack made of baker's yeast and milk is refining.

Soak cotton wool in milk and use as a skin freshener.

Oatmeal

This is another great beauty aid.

For blackheads Rub with oatmeal and water. Rinse with cold water.

Make up a face mask with oatmeal, egg white and a drop of spirits of camphor. Leave the mask on the face for 15 minutes. Remove with luke warm water.

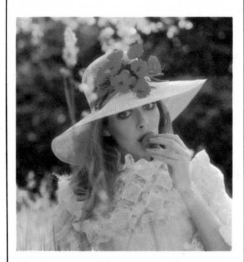

Strawberries, like many other fresh fruits and vegetables, can be used to make deliciously beautifying face masks, tonics and creams

Oatmeal and honey is a good mask for dry skin.

For softening the bath water use a cotton bag filled with oatmeal.

Olive oil

Good for your face, hair and body, particularly for combating dryness. A tablespoon of oil in your bath water will help to stop your suntan fading. Warm olive oil, massaged into the hair and scalp is a superb conditioner immediately before a shampoo.

Before a manicure Soak your finger nails in a small bowl of warm olive oil: it will be good for ragged cuticles.

Oranges

Cover pieces of orange peel in boiled water. Stand. Cool and use the liquid as a skin tonic.

Scratch the fresh peel with a knife to release the orange oil and rub over your arms and neck to make skin more velvety.

Peaches

Peaches, like melons, make a good skin beautifier. Rub slices of the fresh fruit over the face, or put them between layers of gauze and use as a compress for the face.

Potato

Use potato to soften and whiten skin and also to soothe puffiness round the eyes.

Cut a raw potato into slices and rub over your face, neck and hands.

Grate raw potato and place between layers of gauze. Put slices over the eyes and relax for 15 minutes.

Massage hot, tired feet with raw peeled slices of potato. Let the juice dry. Rinse away with tepid water.

Salt

Rub coarse salt into rough skin before bathing. Massage it into the scalp gently as a treatment for dandruff before shampooing.

Strawberries

This fruit is both delicious and beautifying. Mash fresh strawberries and rub over your skin — they are said to lighten it.

Make up a face mask with strawberries, lemon juice and cream.

Mash strawberries to press out the juice and smooth this on to oily skin every day for two weeks.

Tea

Lie down with cold wet teabags on your eyes for half an hour: you will find it very soothing. Another good eye freshener is a mixture of weak tea and rose water. Soak cotton wool in this and pat your eyelids gently.

A hair rinse Cold (milkless) tea.

Tomatoes

Mix the juice of a ripe tomato with equal amounts of lemon juice and glycerine and massage into your hands.

For open pores Put slices of tomato over your face for 15 minutes, and use the time to lie down and relax, too.

Wheatgerm

Wheatgerm oil can be added to face masks or used with other oils for dry hair and skin.

Yogurt

This has many beauty uses. A famous recipe is for a yogurt-and-mint mask. Mix 1 tablespoon of natural yogurt and 1 tablespoon of fuller's earth with a teaspoon of mint (freshly chopped or dried). Apply this to the face (keeping away from the eyes). Leave on for 15 minutes. Wash off.

Yogurt is good for unmanageable hair. Massage it through the hair for 3 minutes, then rinse it off with tepid water.

Use yogurt as a face mask and to smooth over hands and legs. Cooling, softening, whitening, refreshing: yogurt is a good food for beauty.

why eat well?

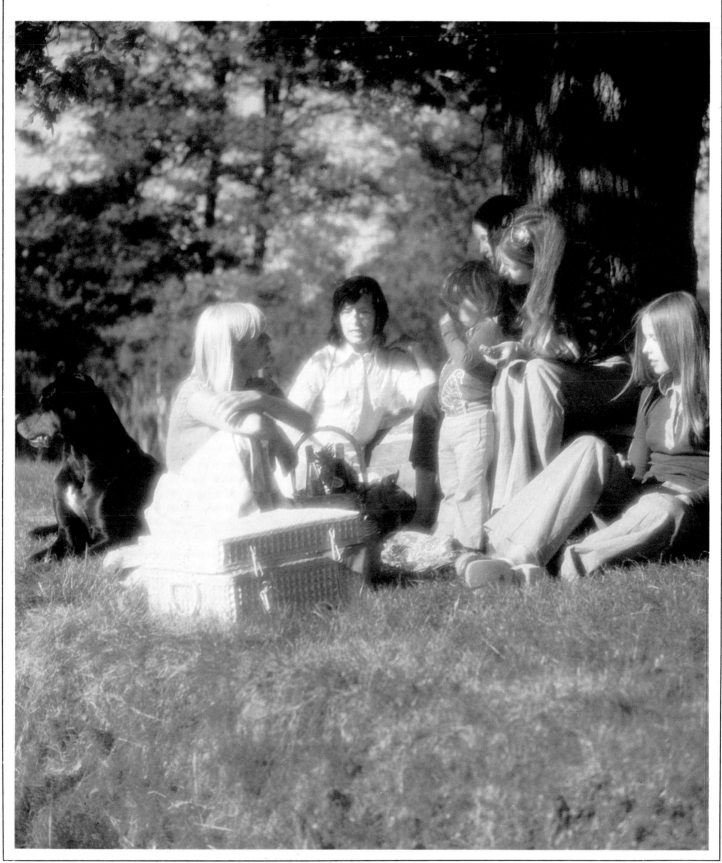

Health, happiness and good looks; all three have far more to do with the food we eat than most of us realize. A healthy diet can be the key to a lifetime of vitality and well-being, and the results of a new attitude to eating are really spectacular:

Good looks. Hair, skin, teeth and eyes can all benefit from an improved diet. And once the correct balance is obtained—excess carbohydrate and sugar being removed—there is certain to be an improvement in the figure too!

Improved health. The addition of vital vitamins and nutrients to a diet which was previously deficient in some ways, can make a big difference to the way you feel. This is particularly noticeable with those minor, nagging ailments—tiredness, irritability, constant colds, headaches.

More energy. Sluggishness and lack of energy can often be traced to some kind of diet deficiency. Irregular, badly-planned meals can lead to constipation, too. If life is beginning to be too much for you, if you never seem able to cope, then think seriously about changing your eating habits. It is so simple to add those missing 'vitality' ingredients to meals. Sometimes, just one basic change (eating more citrus fruits, for example, to step up your quota of vitamin C) can make all the difference to your life.

Better digestion. If you exist on a bland diet of over-refined foods for days and then suddenly indulge in a grand splurge at an exotic restaurant you can expect your stomach to complain. Keep your digestive system working properly all the time, with plenty of roughage—fibrous, bulky foods like bread, bran, wheat germ, raw or dried fruit and green 'stringy' vegetables which help food particles on their way. Then your system will be better able to cope with the unexpected.

None of this means that you have to be faddy about food. What it does mean is that you need the basic nutritional knowledge to enable you to select the best possible foods from the vast choice available. It is more useful to know what to choose from your supermarket shelf than it is to understand the differences between organic and intensive farming methods.

Basic, everyday family menu-planning is more important than preparing a grand dinner party. Day-to-day food is what actually keeps the family in top form; so it's just as important to make sure that you cook food in a way which does not kill all the goodness before it reaches the table as it is to be able to make it look appetizing.

Nutritional know-how

Because eating is a social pastime as well as a basic necessity it is sometimes difficult to relate food intake to actual body chemistry. A delicious cheese soufflé which melts on the tongue may sound positively dreary if broken down into its constituents: protein, carbohydrate, fat, vitamins A, B and E. And if this is followed by a description of what these constituents actually do when they get inside the body, then the whole thing can begin to sound like a chemistry lesson. But you do need to know the basic nutritional facts so that you can relate them to your shopping, menu-planning and cooking methods.

The recipes

All these basic facts are included here. And to help you to use this information in practical ways there are recipes associated with each particular food. (For example, recipes where honey is an important ingredient follow immediately after the information about honey.)

As a further visual guide each recipe has the following symbols:

⧖ This is a guide to the preparation and cooking time required for each dish and will vary according to the skill of the individual cook.

⧖ Less than 1 hour

⧖ ⧖ Between 1 hour and 2½ hours

⧖ ⧖ ⧖ Over 2½ hours

☆ This indicates that the recipe requires no cooking

How to read the charts

Charts which set out the nutritional values of foods are included throughout. The weight measurement used for all the foods in these charts is 100 grams. The amounts of protein, fat and carbohydrate contained in the foods are expressed in grams (g.). The minerals and vitamins in milligrams (mg.). (There are 1000 milligrams to a gram.) So looking at the flour chart (see page 126) you can see, for example, that for every 100 grams of wholemeal [wholewheat] bread you eat you get 8.2 grams of protein and 261 milligrams of potassium.

The only exceptions are vitamins A and D which are commonly expressed in 'International Units'. This is a form of measurement devised by the World Health Organisation and used in this way all over the world.

Remember too that some foods are very much heavier than others. An average portion of, say, Cheddar cheese usually weighs 100 grams and would therefore supply approximately the same nutrients as those mentioned in the chart. However, few people would eat 100 grams of honey at one sitting and you should take this into account when relating the information from the charts to your daily diet.

Thought for food

It makes sense to think about what you eat and make sure you get enough of the essential nutrients. Good food well-cooked not only tastes better than convenience foods but, because it gives your body those nutrients it needs to stay in peak condition, it also makes you look and feel better.

Food deterioration

What makes food 'go off'? Here are some of the things that could speed up the deterioration of food, and some hints on how to avoid them.

Bacteria

These are the most dangerous food contaminators because they can multiply at alarming rates. Although food may have been perfectly safe when it was purchased, it can become dangerously infected by certain disease-carrying bacteria within a few hours. Gastro-enteritis, food poisoning and mild intestinal troubles can usually be traced to bacteria in food, so be very careful. Never keep a meal warm for too long.

Enzymes

These are the catalysts within food which help chemical changes to take place when it is exposed to air and sunlight. Enzymes hasten the destruction of vitamins A and C in fruit and vegetables which are exposed to the air. The only remedy is to make sure that the produce is eaten quickly once it is ripe.

Yeasts

These attack sugary foods—fruit dishes, yogurt, puddings. They give that 'fizzy' taste to the food which although not harmful, is unpleasant. Do not leave sugary dishes in a warm room, or keep them for a long period in a refrigerator. (Yeasts are, of course, deliberately included in home-brewing and baking. But that's a different thing!)

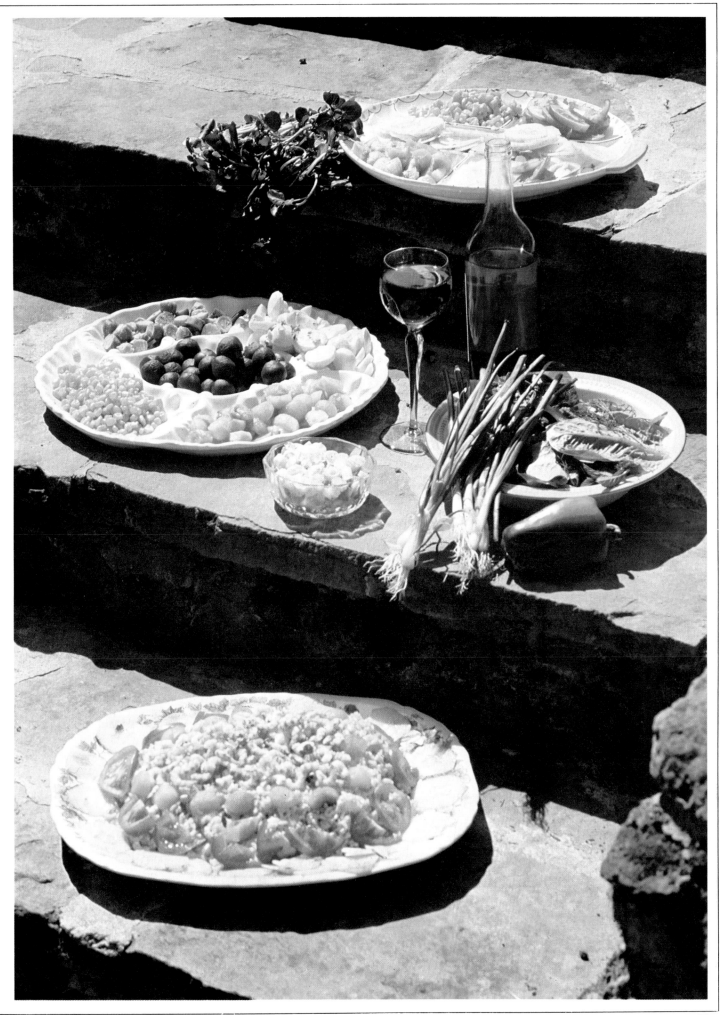

food-what you need, & why

You are what you eat. This may be a simplification of the complicated processes which regulate body metabolism but even so it is basically true. Every cell in the body is made and replaced by constituents derived from the food you eat. The calcium in milk really does make and keep healthy bones and teeth, the iron in vegetables and meat really is responsible for forming healthy red blood cells.

The body is continually repairing itself, so the right kind of food is vital even for adults. And in the process of growing the right nutrients are essential to ensure healthy development.

Eating in the West is a social habit, not a daily bid for survival; most people find it difficult to appreciate the importance of the complicated process of eating which also has important emotional and psychological connections. We eat for comfort; to allay fears; to assuage guilt; because we are happy or because we are sad. These motivations can also affect the kind of food we eat—and we may choose the wrong kind.

Body metabolism

The process by which oxygen is used to convert food into energy is called the metabolic process. To understand metabolism in simple terms, imagine a series of rooms each with a connecting door to the next room. Inside each 'room' chemical changes take place involving various constituents supplied by food. Once the change has taken place, the door to the next 'room' will open satisfactorily. But it will only open if all the constituents were present. In other words, a missing mineral or a missing vitamin in the diet can impede normal metabolism. The door to that 'room' stays firmly shut, and there is a brief—or long-term—breakdown in the process.

Such a breakdown would manifest itself in something minor like splitting nails or something major like anaemia. A vegan diet, for example, comes exclusively from plant and vegetable foods and sometimes results in a lack of vitamin B12. This could lead to severe illness if the vitamin is not supplied as a supplement, for B12 is essential for building and maintaining healthy blood corpuscles.

Energy

As well as the nutrients required for growth and repair, the body also needs energy. The muscles need energy to contract and make the body work. The most important muscle of all is, of course, the heart. It pumps blood around the body. And blood carries the nutrients (taken from food) which will form and renew body cells. Then there are the muscles which control the digestive system; the nerve cells which send signals to the brain; the glands, and all the other parts of the body which have to make or do something in order to keep us alive need energy. Energy is measured in calories. Some foods supply more calories than others. Some people need more calories than others depending on their size, job (i.e. physical and mental activity) and metabolism.

Roughly half the total daily calorie intake is needed for the metabolic processes described above, the rest for physical activities and warmth. Where a person consumes food supplying more calories than he or she requires these are either 'burnt off' by a self-regulating effect of the metabolism or deposited as fat. If a person consumes food supplying fewer calories than he or she needs, the body will make up the amount needed by using fat stored. This is not harmful so long as the food which is consumed supplies the essential nutrients.

High protein Foods
A man in a moderately active job needs about 75 grams of protein a day, and a woman needs about 60. For children, the requirements vary from about 20 grams for a year-old baby, to about 70 for an active teenage boy. (Many doctors are worried that too much protein is introduced too soon into babies' diets. So check the amount required for your baby with your doctor. Young babies get all the protein they need from milk.)

Most people build their meals around the high-protein foods: meat, fish, or (in the case of vegetarians), nuts. The chart below lists 20 top protein-supplying foods. It shows the grams of protein supplied per 100 grams of the food concerned, plus grams for an average portion.

Food	Grams of protein per 100 grams of food	Grams of protein per average portion
Almonds	20.5	about 10 grams for a small handful
Bacon, gammon, fried	31.3	about 16 grams for two rashers
Beef steak, stewed	30.8	about 30 grams for an average serving
Cheese, Cheddar	25.4	about 23 grams for a 3 x 3 x 1 inch square
Cheese, Cottage	16.0	about 18 grams for a small tub or carton
Cheese, Gruyère	37.6	about 30 grams for a 3 x 3 x 1 inch square
Cheese, processed	23.0	about 4 grams for a standard portion
Chicken, roast	29.6	about 25 grams for an average serving
Cod, grilled	27.0	
Crab	19.2	about 4 grams for an average serving
Eggs, fresh, whole	11.9	about 7 grams for a medium-sized egg
Lentils, boiled	6.8	about 3 grams for a tablespoonful
Liver, Calf, fried	29.0	about 25 grams for an average serving
Milk, fresh, whole	3.4	about 9 grams for a large glass (½ pint)
Peanuts	28.1	about 16 grams for a small handful
Peas, split, boiled	8.3	about 5 grams for a tablespoonful
Pork chops, grilled,	25.3	about 5 grams for an average serving
Prawns, boiled	21.2	about 5 grams for an average serving
Sardines, canned	20.4	about 6 grams for a small tub or carton
Yogurt, low fat	4.7	

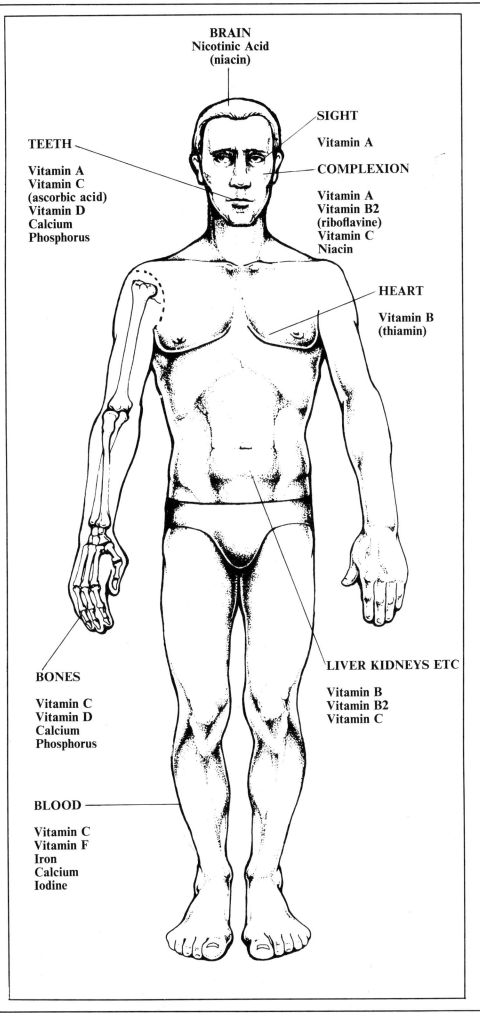

BRAIN
Nicotinic Acid
(niacin)

SIGHT

Vitamin A

COMPLEXION

Vitamin A
Vitamin B2
(riboflavine)
Vitamin C
Niacin

TEETH

Vitamin A
Vitamin C
(ascorbic acid)
Vitamin D
Calcium
Phosphorus

HEART

Vitamin B
(thiamin)

LIVER KIDNEYS ETC

Vitamin B
Vitamin B2
Vitamin C

BONES

Vitamin C
Vitamin D
Calcium
Phosphorus

BLOOD

Vitamin C
Vitamin F
Iron
Calcium
Iodine

Vitamins and minerals

We tend to talk glibly about the importance of vitamins and minerals without considering just how recently the function of these substances was discovered. For up until the end of the nineteenth century very little work had been done to isolate the biochemical actions of the nutrients in foods. In 1753 James Lind recommended that scurvy should be treated by including lemons in the diet. This recommendation was based on observation; he did not know that citrus fruits contain vitamin C, and that scurvy is caused by vitamin C deficiency.

The word 'vitamine' was coined by a Swiss scientist named Casimir Funk at the beginning of the twentieth century. He based the name on the assumption that all these vital factors were nitrogen-containing substances called 'amines'. Later this was found to be untrue, so the 'e' was dropped from the name.

Much work is still to be done on the exact function of vitamins in the body. And research still needs to be carried out to discover just how these minute organic substances can be used in treating disease. Researches now indicate, for example, that there is a link between lack of vitamin E and heart disease. And the vitamin B complex, which contains more than 15 different substances, is also the subject of a great deal of research—particularly because the main source (the whole germ of wheat) is rapidly disappearing from Western diet.

The mineral substances in food are equally vital for in many cases they actually trigger off the action of the vitamins. Again, their importance is only just being fully realized, particularly that of the 'trace' minerals. Although these are only present in foods in minute quantities, they are essential to health. The removal of these minerals from foods during refining processes is causing much concern.

The charts over list the most important vitamins and minerals together with their functions and best food sources.

THE PRINCIPAL VITAMINS

Common name	Chemical name(s)	Good sources	Daily needs	What it does for you	Discovery date
A	Retinol	Fish liver oils, animal liver, eggs, milk, yogurt, butter, green leafy vegetables, carrots.	2.7 mg	Essential for body growth and proper function of the retina. Helps resistance to infections.	1913
B1	Thiamine, aneurine	Yeast, wheat germ, wholemeal wholewheat flour, lean meat.	1.2 mg	Essential factor in carbohydrate metabolism. Important for nervous system, digestive system and heart. Severe lack causes beriberi whick can lead to heart failure and damage to the nervous system.	1936
B2	Riboflavin	Yeast, wheat germ, liver, kidneys, cheese, meat.	1.7 mg	Important for normal growth of skin, nails and hair. Deficiency causes dull hair, split fingernails, itching eyes.	1933
B6	Pyridoxine	Yeast, wheat germ, liver, potatoes.	1.5 mg	For healthy skin and proper growth in children.	1936
	Niacin nicotinic acid,	Yeast, wheat, bread, liver, meat, fish, chicken, mushrooms.	19 mg	For healthy skin (anti-pellagra), mucous membranes and nervous system.	1937
(H)	Biotin	Yeast, peanuts, peas, mushrooms.	Unknown	Uncertain	1940
	Pantothenic acid	Yeast, liver, beans, mushrooms, peanuts.	Unknown	Uncertain	1938
	Folic acid	Yeast, liver, milk, green vegetables.	0.15 mg	Healthy blood	1944
B12	Cyanocobalamin	Liver, meat, wholemeal (wholewheat) flour, wheat germ.	0.005 mg	Healthy blood. This is known as the anti-pernicious anaemia vitamin.	1948
C	Ascorbic acid	Fresh fruit and vegetables especially citrus fruits, blackcurrants, tomatoes, rosehips.	30 mg	Vitality, resistance to infections, helps the body to resist shock, too. Essential for the formation of the body 'cement' which holds together the inter-cellular material making up the connective tissue, bones, teeth and blood-vessel walls.	1928
D	Calciferol	Fish liver oils, eggs, milk, butter, sunshine on skin.	0.01 mg	Regulates calcium and phosphorous content of the body. (This is essential in teeth and bone formation). Mostly needed during childhood but essential, too, during pregnancy.	1922
E	Tocopherol	Wheat germ, whole grains, nuts, vegetable oils.	Unknown	Protects body tissues. Keeps blood circulating freely.	1923
K		Green vegetables, liver, tomatoes, carrot tops, soya bean oil, seaweed.	Unknown	Essential for maintenance of prothrombin, one of the blood-clotting factors in blood plasma. Therefore helps to heal wounds.	1935

THE PRINCIPAL MINERALS

Common name	Chemical name	Good sources	What it does for you
Calcium	Ca	Milk, cheese, sardines or other small fish eaten whole with bones, parsley, watercress, molasses.	All body cells need calcium. Essential for the formation of bones, teeth, hair, fingernails. Protects the nervous system, helps blood clotting and is important in maintaining healthy body fluids, membrane and muscles. Particularly vital for growing children and pregnant women. (Calcium needs vitamin D to aid absorption).
Cobalt	Co	Sweetbreads, mushrooms, liver.	Constituent of vitamin B12 and concerned with the promotion of healthy nerve fibres and tissues of the bone Guards against types of anaemia.
Copper	Cu	Liver, kidney, egg yolk, lentils, wholemeal (wholewheat) flour, parsley, brown sugar, brazil nuts and walnuts.	Concerned with several enzyme systems including those responsible for the oxidation of vitamin C.
Fluorine	F	Drinking water in certain areas, seafoods, tea (particularly China tea).	Builds up tooth enamel in children and guards against tooth decay.
Iodine	I	Seafoods, Kelp, sea salt. Fruit, vegetables and cereals may contain supplies but amounts vary depending on area.	Essential for correct functioning of the thyroid gland, guards against goitre, keeps body cells and circulation active. Also assists in healthy development of the brain and continuing sexual interest.
Iron	Fe	Egg yolk, liver, black pudding (blood sausage), molasses, corned beef, peanuts, lentils and some green vegetables (e.g. watercress).	Helps make blood. During child-bearing years women need more iron than men (they lose large amounts during menstruation). Iron is also concerned with the formation of body cells and production of energy. Deficiency may cause anaemia.
Magnesium	Mg	Green salads, green vegetables, nuts, beans, lentils, whole grains.	Concerned with strength and well-being of bones, teeth, nerves, muscles, hair and nails.
Manganese	Mn	Liver, kidney, beans, lentils, cereals, tea and coffee, nuts.	Activator in a number of enzyme systems. A deficiency in animals produces poor growth and reproduction, and occasional anaemia. It can also cause bone changes and disturbances in the central nervous system and a disappearance of sexual drive.
Phosphorus	P	Milk, cheese, egg yolk, yeast, wholemeal (wholewheat) flour, nuts, meat.	Helps make bones, teeth, body cells and tissues, hair and fingernails. Helps the release of energy during the processing of carbohydrates. Phosphorus needs vitamin D to assist absorption. Many of the B group of vitamins work only when combined with phosphates in the body.
Potassium	K	Dried apricots, beans, nuts, dried currants, dates, figs, grapes, prunes, raisins, sultanas, soya flour, molasses, yeast, brown sugar.	Works with sodium to maintain a correct fluid balance. Essential for heart rhythm, nerve activity and the processing of carbohydrates.
Selenium	Se	Liver, kidney, heart.	Acts with vitamin E to maintain a healthy condition of the liver and also to inhibit the development of muscular dystrophy.
Sodium	Na	Dried apricots, beans, nuts, table salt, ham, bread, beef extract, celery, eggs, spinach,	Acts with potassium to correct fluid balance.
Sulphur	S	Nuts, dried fruits, oatmeal, barley, beans, cheese, meat,	Helps in the construction and maintenance of body cells and muscle fibres.
Zinc	Z	Oysters, sweetbreads, liver.	Involved in several enzyme systems and constituent of insulin. Eyes, teeth and testes all contain considerable amounts.

eating for health & beauty

Eating well will make the very best of your looks and could certainly help to prevent certain kinds of ill-health. Skin, hair and figure are all important beauty areas. All three need the right nutrients to look really good, and the right nutrients are supplied by food. Colds, influenza and depression are common ailments, and they can be 'treated' with food.

This deceptively simple-sounding theory can, perhaps, be best illustrated by an extreme example. Imagine two 20-year-old girls, both working as secretaries, both with 'average' characteristics: brown hair, brown eyes, slightly 'pear-shaped' figure, medium height, fairly slow-working, sluggish metabolism.

Girl A eats well. Her diet consists of fresh fruit, vegetables (good for skin, hair and figure), lean meat, fish, dairy foods and salads. She always eats a reasonably good breakfast, and takes her meals at regular times. When she goes out to dinner and eats more than usual, she restricts her carbohydrate intake the next day and eats more fruit. She drinks water, milk, a little tea and coffee and a little alcohol.

This girl looks good. Her figure is firm and trim, her face is spot-free, her hair is glossy. She has vitality and an outgoing personality. She feels good, too. Her teeth are in good shape, she gets the occasional cold, but soon shakes it off, and common ailments do not often trouble her.

Girl B eats badly. Her diet consists of snack foods: fried meals, sandwiches, cakes, confectionery, plus the occasional tray meal. She eats few fresh vegetables and little fruit. She drinks sugar-loaded soft drinks and quite a bit of alcohol. She eats very little during the day—except fattening nibbles—and has lots of fried foods during the evening. She takes little exercise.

This girl is not doing herself justice. Her skin is spotty due to lack of vitamins B and C, her hair is lank and her figure is spreading. Her teeth seem to be more 'filling' than enamel (the sugary foods attract caries-forming bacteria), and she feels sluggish and depressed. She also seems to be a sitting target for all minor diseases. Last winter, she was in bed with influenza for three weeks and then had a succession of colds. She feels too tired to bother about her appearance or her work. Her doctor says that overweight could lead to high blood pressure.

Girl A is obviously making the most of herself, Girl B isn't. Even a natural beauty would have problems staying beautiful on B's diet. At best, she would feel sluggish and below par, at worst she would have dull hair, an unattractively spotty face and a lumpy figure.

Give your body a chance to prove how good it can look and feel. Provide it with the fuel, in the form of good food, to keep ticking over nicely.

General health

Minimize the chances of succumbing to germs by making sure that your resistance is not low. Keep up your vitamin C level by eating oranges, grapefruit and green vegetables every day for vitamin C cannot be stored by the body. Doctors are concerned that modern eating habits seem to be tending to exclude sufficient quantities of the vitamin B complex. Make sure you get enough of these by drinking plenty of milk, and eating lean meat, liver, fish and some wheat germ and brewer's yeast.

Weight

Overweight really can lead to illness. Ailments which strike fat people more than lean people include heart troubles, diabetes, cerebral haemorrhage, digestive complaints and impotence. So adopting a good, well-balanced diet which is low in calories and high in essential nutrients is clearly a sensible idea.

Looks

Skin needs vitamin B2. This is present in fresh vegetables, milk and wholemeal [wholewheat] bread. Skin also needs vitamin C to purify and vitalize the blood-stream. Eat at least one orange a day, or take vitamin C supplement.

Teeth and bones need calcium and vitamin D. These are found in milk, fish oils (and the small edible bones in sardines) and yeast. Keep teeth in super health by cleaning regularly and avoiding the caries-encouraging sugary foods.

Hair is made from a protein-based substance called keratin so it needs protein and the B vitamins. (Hospitals give high protein diets to patients who have lost body hair through accidents.) A high protein diet can help your hair to grow strongly. Fish, meat, cheese, eggs and offal are all good for your hair. Yeast taken as a supplement in tablet form can also help.

Nails need protein (they, too, are keratin based), plus minerals like iodine.

Eyes need vitamin A to help to retina to function properly and to prevent night-blindness. Drink lots of water to help eyes sparkle, and eat carrots, cabbage and other green leafy vegetables, butter, eggs and fish liver oils. Avoid alcohol or stimulants like coffee and tea. These can cause red, dull eyes.

Eating for prevention and cure
Listed below are some common ailments and beauty problems, plus the foods which could help to prevent and cure them. But seek the advice of your doctor too.

Ailment or problem	Foods which can help—and why	Ailment or problem	Foods which can help—and why
Common cold, influenza.	Massive doses of vitamin C have been recommended both as treatment and a preventative—two or three oranges a day, plus plenty of raw green vegetables.	Sluggish metabolism, goitre, sluggish thyroid	These are all related to thyroid gland secretion, and this depends on sufficient iodine—found in seafoods, iodized salt and kelp.
Acne.	Vitamins B and C help to keep skin clear. If your skin is blotchy and tired-looking, drink lots of water, eat citrus fruits and green vegetables	Lethargy, pale skin, anaemia.	Iron is vital for the formation of red blood cells which carry oxygen to all parts of the body. About a quarter of all women are iron-deficient. Eat liver, kidney or heart.
		Falling hair, brittle nails.	You need protein to build keratin, hair follicles and nails, together with sulphur and vitamins B and D to keep them healthy. Eat meat, fish, cheese, eggs, cabbage.
Constipation, gastro-enteritis.	Natural yogurt can help to soothe troubled stomachs and ward off infection.	Depression, insomnia.	Vitamin B1 (thiamine), B2 (riboflavin) and protein can help. Brewer's yeast is a good source.

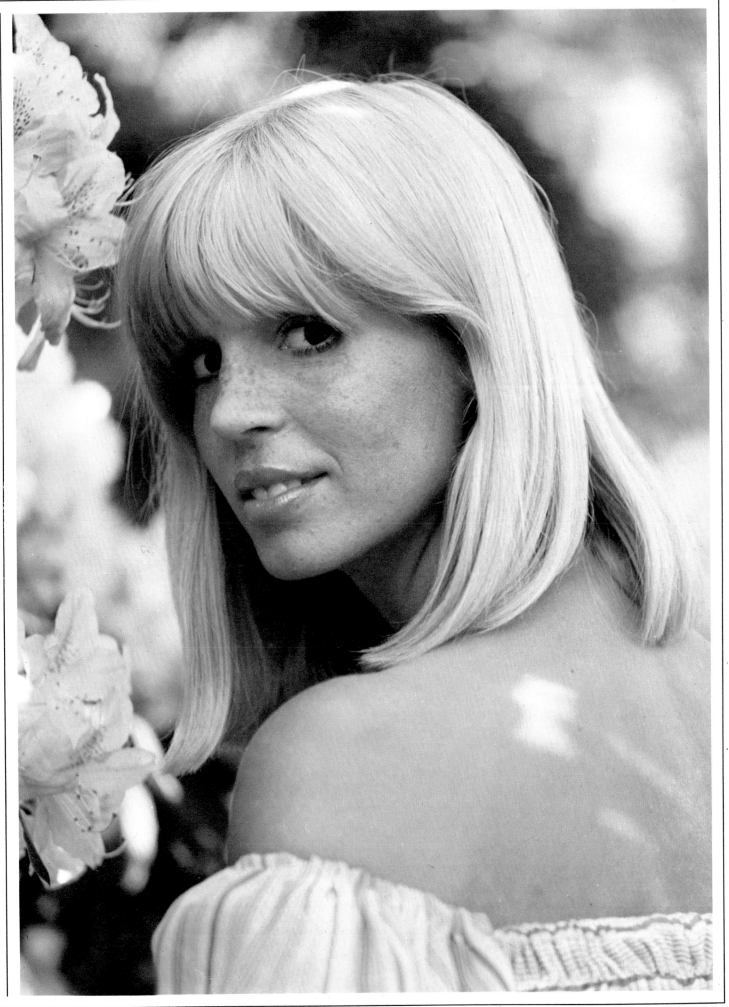

food & sexuality

Healthy eating really can improve your sex life by providing the nutrients, vitamins and minerals which give you a desire for sexual fulfilment plus the energy and stamina to enjoy it. It may come as a surprise to know that most so-called 'aphrodisiac' foods really do contribute vital substances which play an important part in desire and fertility. These foods will not produce an overnight result, but taken regularly they can have a marked effect.

Take the 'myth' about the aphrodisiac powers of oysters, for example. Apparently, Casanova considered oysters to be so potent that he ate about 50 a day. Chemically, he could have been on to a good thing because oysters are a rich source of zinc, which encourages healthy growth and guards against anaemia. The eyes, teeth and testes all contain considerable amounts of zinc. Other traditional aphrodisiac foods—mushrooms, radishes (used as a sex food by the ancient Egyptians) and watercress—are less expensive than oysters and probably just as effective. There is no need to splurge on caviar and artichokes to guarantee a lifetime of love. A good diet of fresh and homely foods like salads, green vegetables and the cheaper cuts of meat are just as good. Even a weekly meal which includes liver —rich in vitamins A, B1, B2 and E— a salad and some fresh fruit will help to keep you sexually active. The essence of a virile body is a good diet.

Stamina

Up to 50 per cent of all women experience iron-deficiency at some time

Aphrodisiacs—fact or fiction?

Some well-known and not-so-well-known 'aphrodisiac' foods are listed below—plus a few good reasons why they may actually work!

Eggs
Iron, protein, vitamins A, B and E, phosphorus and copper are all supplied by eggs.

Oysters
These contain zinc which is present in eyes, teeth and testes, encourages healthy growth and discourages anaemia. Zinc also helps to keep skin young and supple and a deficiency can cause premature ageing.
(Zinc is also found in sweetbreads and liver.)

Liver and kidney
These may not seem romantic foods but they should be added to the list as they contain minerals like copper, manganese, zinc and iron—all of which help to stimulate sexual urges—together with vitamins A, B, C and E.

Saffron, cinnamon, pepper, peppermint, ginger
These spices that tempt the palate are also generally supposed to tempt the sexual appetite. To date, however, there is no evidence to show why they should.

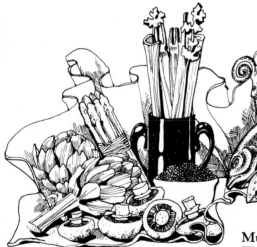

Lobsters
Iodine is the 'life tempo' mineral which keeps body cells healthy and aids circulation. It also helps to keep you young and thinking about sex. Because they contain iodine lobsters are a good choice for health and sex-conscious businessmen. But, if lobster is too expensive, haddock, herring and whiting are effective substitutes.

Mushrooms
These contain vitamins B1 and B2 plus a good sprinkling of minerals. Truffles have the same qualities, and have long been trusted as an effective aphrodisiac.

Caviar
Any fish roe is an excellent source of potassium—for muscular strength, mental clarity, vitality—and other vital minerals. Cod's roe is just as good if caviar is too expensive.

Asparagus, celery, artichokes
These three vegetables are often quoted as aphrodisiacs. Certainly they are good sources of vitamins B and C, and stimulate taste buds and digestive juices. Celery is probably the most versatile, and the least expensive, of the three.

during their child-bearing years. (The worst times of all are just before and after menstruation.) Iron-deficiency makes you feel 'droopy' and below par, so an iron supplement in food or tablet form is vital if you want to stay in top form throughout each month. Meat, green vegetables—particularly watercress—and offal [variety meats] will help.

Protein is good for stamina, too. So eat lots of meat, eggs, cheese and fish.

Fertility

It has been shown that obesity can impede fertility in both men and women. Solve your weight problem and you could go a long way towards solving your fertility one, too. Quite apart from the biological factors involved, being seriously overweight is aesthetically undesirable for a full, rewarding sex-life. So fresh, lightly-cooked food is infinitely better than heavy carbohydrate-packed 'stodge' if you want to maintain a healthy interest in sex for as long as possible. Middle-age spread is a strong anti-love-making factor—keep a firm, reasonably slim body and you will keep your love-life active.

Virility

Go to bed on a full stomach at your peril. A heavy meal eaten late at night will slow down desire and responses to love-making. Nowadays, there is a tendency to eat the main meal of the day half-way through the evening, sometimes hunched over a tray watching television at the same time. This is unfortunate because both digestion and love-life can suffer. A full stomach, especially if accompanied by the effects of alcohol, will induce drowsiness.

A woman who has eaten earlier in the evening and who is ready for love at bedtime can hardly expect her man to show the same enthusiasm if she has just presented him with a huge cooked meal or a pile of sandwiches. If you must serve—or eat—a late meal make it light: a tossed salad and cold meat or fish, a slice of wholemeal [wholewheat] bread and fruit to follow. Avoid heavy sauces, pasta, potatoes, stodgy puddings and spirits.

Milky drinks are sleep-inducing, too. Why not try an energy-inducing nightcap for a change? Mix 3 tablespoons natural yogurt, 8 tablespoons freshly-squeezed orange juice, 2 tablespoons honey, 1 teaspoon apple cider vinegar and a sprinkling of wheat germ flakes. Stir and drink. It tastes surprisingly good and it does you good too.

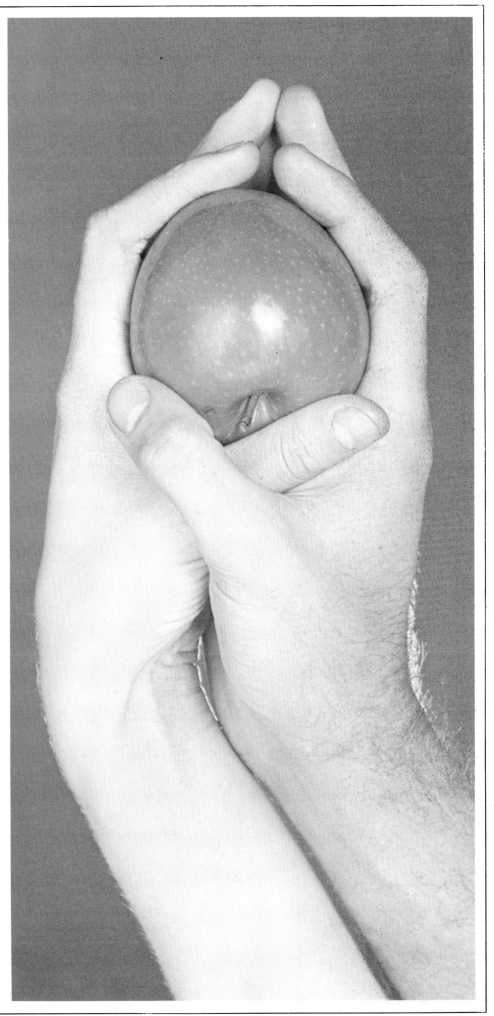

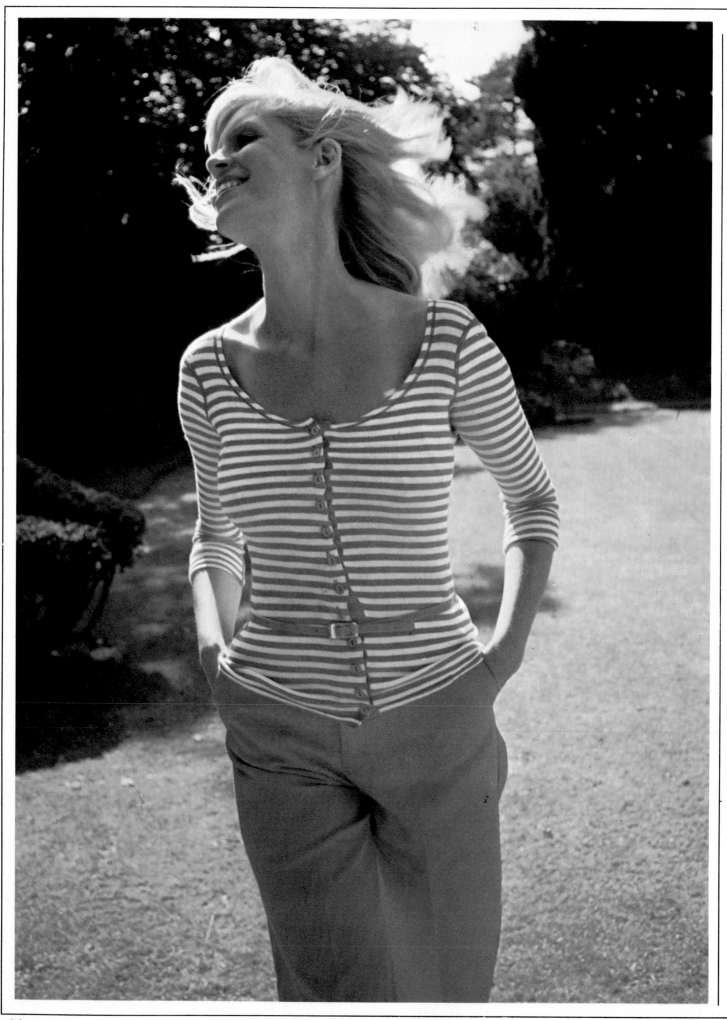

vitality diet

This one-week diet plan provides all the nutrients required for good health and good looks. Use it as a tonic when you feel below par, or when you know that your food intake has been badly balanced over the past few weeks.

Follow this diet exactly for just one week. You will find yourself feeling so much better that you will resolve to keep up the good food habits you have acquired.

Avoid alcohol during the day, but do sip mead* or wine with the evening meal, or beer if you prefer it. Spirits should be avoided when possible.

At the beginning of the diet we give you suggestions for mid-morning and mid-afternoon snacks to keep you feeling at top form when energy is flagging. After two days, however, you should feel able to go through from breakfast to lunch and lunch to the evening meal without a snack.

If you do feel hungry between meals have a piece of fresh fruit or a glass of fruit juice. This will effectively raise a flagging blood-sugar level without adding the pure sucrose found in sweets, cakes and buns.

Day One
Breakfast:
Fresh, unsweetened orange juice
2 tablespoons Muesli* with milk
1 slice wholemeal [wholewheat] bread*
  with a little butter and honey
Decaffeinated coffee with milk, no sugar

Mid-morning:
1 glass vegetable juice* (choose any one of the recipes)

Lunch:
Cottage cheese lunch platter*
1 banana
Large glass milk

Mid-afternoon:
1 orange

Evening meal:
Chicken with tarragon sauce*
Buttered spinach
1 slice wholemeal [wholewheat] bread*
  with a little butter
Fig and apple pie*

Day Two
Breakfast:
Unsweetened tomato juice with 1 teaspoon wheat germ stirred in
1 egg, boiled, with 1 slice bran bread and butter
1 orange
Decaffeinated coffee with milk, no sugar

Mid-morning:
1 dish yogurt* mixed with dried fruit (raisins, chopped apricots, etc.)

Lunch:
Lemon consommé with yogurt*
Cottage cheese and mushroom quiche*
Bean salad*
Large glass milk

Mid-afternoon:
1 glass vegetable juice (choose any one of the recipes)

Evening meal:
Baked cod* with watercress dressing*
Date and orange salad*
1 slice banana nut bread* with a little butter

Day Three
Breakfast:
Yogurt with orange whip*
1 slice wholemeal [wholewheat] bread*
  with a little butter and honey
Decaffeinated coffee with milk, no sugar.

Lunch:
Onion soup*
Braised beef rolls with beans*
Small bunch grapes
Large glass orange juice

Evening meal:
Liver with basil*
Green salad
Date and orange salad*

Day Four
Breakfast:
1 dish yogurt* with 1 tablespoon honey and a sprinkling of wheat germ
Compôte of fresh fruit
1 slice wholemeal [wholewheat] bread*
  with a little butter
Decaffeinated coffee with milk, no sugar

Lunch:
Chicken casserole*
Watercress and carrot salad*
1 slice wholemeal [wholewheat] bread*
  with a little butter
1 orange
Tea with lemon

Evening meal:
Pizza with cheese and olives*
Slice of banana nut bread*

Day Five
Breakfast:
1 egg, poached, on 1 slice of wholemeal [wholewheat] bread*, toasted
Stewed prunes
Decaffeinated coffee with milk, no sugar

Lunch:
Clear vegetable soup with cheese and yogurt*
Sliced cold meats with Cole slaw salad*
Honey raisin pudding*
Large glass orange juice

Evening meal:
Baked stuffed mackerel*
Crunchy winter salad with piquant dressing*
1 orange

Day Six
Breakfast:
Unsweetened grapefruit juice
Herb omelette made from 1 egg with mushrooms
1 slice wholemeal [wholewheat] bread*
  with a little butter
Decaffeinated coffee with milk, no sugar

Lunch:
Braised beef rolls with beans*
Coconut apples*
Large glass milk

Evening meal:
Smoked fish and cottage cheese cocottes*
Moroccan vegetable couscous*
Honey biscuits*

Day Seven
Breakfast:
Unsweetened tomato juice with 1 teaspoon wheat germ stirred in
1 egg, boiled, with 1 slice bran bread and butter
1 apple
Decaffeinated coffee with milk, no sugar

Lunch:
Avocado rice salad*
1 small piece cheese
Large glass milk

Evening meal:
Brazil nut salad*
Fish fillets, Spanish style*
Crispy salad* with mayonnaise*
Date and orange salad*

how to get the most from food

The way you prepare and cook food is just as important as the way you select it. There is little point in shopping around for the freshest fruit, vegetables and meat and then destroying much of their nutritional value by bad storage, bad preparation and, finally, over-cooking. Many cooks are guilty of all these things, although their meals may be delicious and palatable.

Buying food

Food starts to deteriorate from the moment it leaves its original source. So it is important to buy fresh produce as near that source as possible. Once food is caught up in the warehouse—wholesaler—retailer—consumer process important nutrients can be lost. This is particularly true of fresh fruit and vegetables. Vitamin C is very volatile. Enzymes in the plants themselves cause this vitamin to combine with oxygen in the air, lowering the vitamin level in the plant. So long periods of storage in warehouse or shop mean a poor deal in terms of food-value for the consumer. Growing your own produce is one solution to this problem (see page 128). Alternatively, find a reliable retailer or buy direct the grower.

Food storage

Ideally, food should be stored for as short a time as possible. If you can shop every day so much the better. But many people find it more convenient to shop two or three times a week, or even weekly. In this case, careful storage of fresh food becomes vital. Here is a guide to help you keep it in prime condition.

Fruit and vegetables Store these in a cool, dark place. Light can accelerate the rate at which vitamin C is lost. The enzymes which cause the destruction of vitamins A and C cannot act when the food is chilled so the refrigerator is the ideal place to keep fruit and vegetables. (Produce with heavy peel—bananas, oranges, potatoes—are the exceptions as the peel gives a certain amount of protection from oxygen.) Never keep vegetables in the refrigerator for too long. If you do the moisture in them will start to dry out. And never store fruit and vegetables too close to the freezer section or the moisture will freeze and ruin the produce.

Meat and fish Buy meat and fish as close to the time of consumption as possible. Store it at the top of the refrigerator, near the freezer section. This is particularly vital in the case of offal [variety meats], minced [ground] meat, sausages, all fish and poultry. Anything purchased frozen should be kept frozen until you are going to use it, and then allowed to thaw slowly and thoroughly before cooking. Never cook partly-frozen meat or fish, and never re-freeze it once it has thawed.

Milk and milk products If milk is allowed to stand on the doorstep in sunshine for two hours half its vitamin B2 (riboflavin) content will be destroyed. To preserve nutrients place milk, and milk products such as yogurt and cream, in the refrigerator as quickly as possible; use them the same day if you can.

Eggs Eggs are best used in cooking when they are at room temperature, so it is unnecessary to keep them in the refrigerator. They are a very valuable food. Five eggs a week provide one person with 16 per cent of the recommended intake of vitamin D, 8 per cent of that of vitamin B2 and 7 per cent of that of both iron and vitamin A. These nutrients stay intact while the egg is fresh, so consume eggs quickly. (One word of warning, however: eggs are high in cholesterol which is believed to be linked with some forms of heart disease.)

Bread and flour-based foods Keep bread covered in a dry, cool part of the kitchen. Damp will encourage mould but, on the other hand, a hot, dry atmosphere will make the bread go stale quickly. Do not throw away bread simply because it has become a little dry. Toast it instead. Bread toasted golden brown loses little of its vitamin content and becomes easier to digest.

Other foods Remember that canned and dried foods do not necessarily have an unlimited life. Canned ham and pork products should be used within six months, and no canned food should be kept in damp surroundings which could cause the cans to go rusty. (And never leave food in an opened tin. If you do not use all of it at once put the remainder in a bowl and store it in the refrigerator.)

The same rules apply to dried foods. Excessive moisture could cause the reconstitution of products such as dried peas or dried fruit to begin, and then deterioration could take place in just the same way as it would with the fresh equivalent. Flour, sugar, coffee and tea should always be kept in air-tight containers in a dry, warm place—near the stove, perhaps.

Pots and pans for healthy cooking

Iron cooking pots may have been heavy and difficult to clean, but they did have one distinct advantage: iron-deficiency was largely prevented by people actually eating bits of cooking pot. Iron pots and pans have now largely been replaced by lighter, labour-saving metals which often have a non-stick coating for easy washing. These newer metals have been criticized for possible food-contamination.

Aluminium, for example, is a soft metal which combines with food which is cooked in it or left to stand in it for long periods of time. Two toxins, aluminium hydroxide and aluminium oxide, may then be taken into the system when the food is eaten. Most aluminium pans are meant for quick cooking—boiling vegetables, etc. Use them this way, never leave food standing in them and there is no danger. Flame-proof earthenware pots and casseroles are the best choice for long, slow cooking.

Non-stick coating materials may also be suspect. When the resin coating is heated to high temperatures fumes are released which may be toxic. However, really high temperatures may also damage the surface so it is wise to use these pans on gentle or moderate heat.

Earthenware or non-enamelled iron are the safest materials for casseroles. There is a danger that enamelled

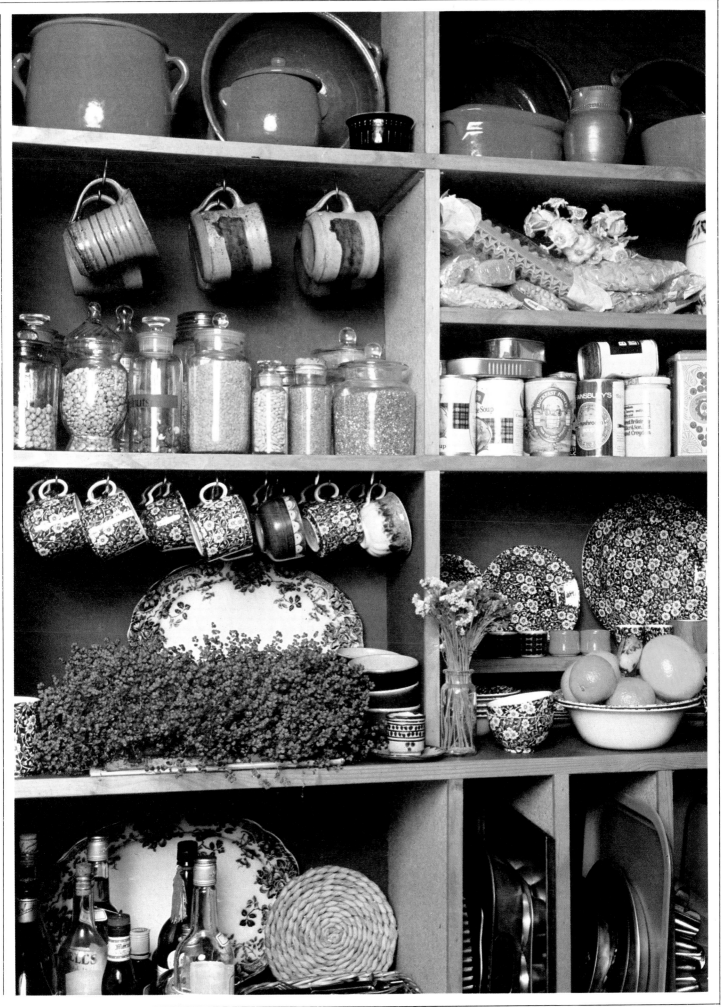

casseroles could contaminate food, especially if the lid is coloured red, yellow or orange or if there is a design on the underside of the lid and the inside of the pot. The coloured enamel used could contain lead or cadmium, and when cooking starts, and the steam condenses inside the pot and under the lid, small quantities of these two poisons could drip into the food. Lead poisoning has been linked with brain damage and cadmium with kidney trouble. But this danger only exists if it is an old pot and food is eaten from it regularly. (Manufacturers have stopped using enamel containing these poisons so this warning does not apply to new casseroles.) If you suspect that one of your cooking pots may be contaminated, use it with greaseproof [waxed] paper or foil under the lid, and throw this away after cooking.

Washing up

It is vital to clean all pans thoroughly after use, particles of old food left in the pan and re-heated when you next use it may encourage bacteria which could spread to the food being freshly cooked.

Wash and clean cutlery properly, paying particular attention to forks which sometimes trap particles of food between the prongs. And do make sure that the cutlery drawer is cleaned regularly. There is no point in putting shining utensils back in a dirty, germ-ridden cupboard.

If you have a dish-washer, clean the filter every day according to the manufacturer's instructions, scrub the racks and cutlery holders from time to time. Finally, clean the sink itself thoroughly at least once a day, sprinkling a good disinfectant down the waste-pipe and drain. Germs love sinks, dish-cloths, dish-mops, scourers and all the associated kitchen paraphernalia.

Food preparation

Paradoxically, an excess of hygiene can be a dangerous thing, particularly in the preparation of food. If this sounds unlikely consider the cook who ruthlessly strips away the outside leaves of vegetables, thoroughly soaks what remains in salted water and perhaps even leaves them in the water until cooking time. Vegetables treated in this way will certainly be clean, but valuable vitamins and minerals will be lost. (Vitamins B and C are soluble in water.) The rule for all food preparation is to be thorough but quick.

Meat Wash meat quickly under a cold tap, dry it thoroughly and then cook it. Never soak meat. Do make sure that frozen meat—particularly chicken—is completely thawed before cooking, but do not leave the thawed meat standing in a warm room for long. Where meat is to be trimmed or cut up for a specific dish try to preserve the blood which drains off as this contains a high proportion of the iron content.

Fish Scrape the scales off both sides of the fish under running water; use a knife and work from the tail towards the head. Remove entrails from round fish by making a slit from the gills half-way to the tail, drawing out the insides and cleaning away any blood. Flat fish, such as sole and plaice [flounder], should be slit through the cavity which lies in the upper part of the body under the gills. Then the entrails can be cleaned out in the same way. Cut off gills, fins, head and tail if desired, rinse quickly again and then cook.

Fruit and vegetables Do not discard peelings and outside leaves on vegetables. If possible, leave them on. Most young green vegetables have tender outside leaves, and these often contain the greatest concentration of nutrients. Never discard the tough ones either. Keep a special bag or pan for carrot, radish and celery tops, pea-pods and the outer leaves of lettuce, cabbage, spinach and cauliflower. These can be the basis of a really good soup stock.

Fruit is best eaten raw, peel and all, but when you intend to cook it remember not to soak it in water beforehand. Fruits which have a thick peel—oranges, grapefruit and lemons—will obviously have to be peeled. But the peel is delicious grated and added to the final dish.

Potatoes and other root vegetables should be washed quickly but thoroughly and, if possible, cooked without being peeled. The peel can be easily removed before serving. The minerals are often concentrated just below the skin and are lost if the vegetable is peeled thickly. (New potatoes are, of course, delicious eaten skin and all.) If you want to prepare vegetables in advance, wash and dry them thoroughly and store them in a plastic bag or container in the refrigerator. Never leave vegetables in a saucepan for hours before you cook them.

Salads Wash salad vegetables quickly in running water and make sure they are dried properly before any dressing is applied. This is necessary for two reasons. First, the dressing will not adhere to the leaves if they are wet. Secondly, valuable vegetable juices could be drawn out into any available moisture when salt is added to the finished dish. Keep salad vegetables in the refrigerator. Never leave them floating in the sink.

Cooking

The shorter the cooking time, the less vitamins are lost. But the way you cook food, and the time it is kept hot before serving, are also vitally important. Large-scale caterers who have to keep food hot for long periods are, probably unwittingly, depriving their customers of nutrients. So if you have to eat in a restaurant or canteen every day, do not rely on those bulk-prepared vegetables for your daily supply of vitamin C.

Boiling It is never a good idea to boil food for long periods. Try to cut down the time that vegetables, meat or fish are boiling in liquid, use a very little water or stock and cover the pan so that vitamins and minerals do not disappear in steam. All minerals, sugars, vitamin C and all the B complex vitamins are soluble in water, even when the food is raw. During boiling all nutrients, including those which do not dissolve in water, will gradually pass into the cooking liquid. Use that cooking liquid to make gravies or broths even if only a few tablespoons are left.

There is a theory that the greatest loss of vitamins from food occurs between the time that the food is put on the heat and the time when it reaches boiling point, so try to shorten this period as much as possible.

Steaming This can help to reduce vitamin loss if it is carefully done. If possible, buy a steamer—a pan with a wire basket inside which holds the vegetables above the water-level in the pan.

If you don't have a steamer however, you can still steam leafy vegetables. Put two or three tablespoons of water into the pan, cover and boil until the pan is filled with steam. The steam will then replace the oxygen which usually destroys vitamins A and C. Add the vegetables quickly, cover the pan again and cook the food as quickly as possible. It is vital that the steam should be kept inside the pan throughout the cooking period. And remember to use any liquid left after cooking for gravies and broths.

'Short' cooking The Chinese and Japanese have this technique down to a fine art, and it is an excellent way of preserving the nutrients in vegetables, meat and fish. Chop the food finely and then cook it quickly in a pan with a little vegetable oil to prevent it sticking. For dinner parties this can be done over a spirit stove at the table.

The only possible disadvantage to this method is that breaking up food does increase the surfaces exposed to oxygen, and so may accelerate the deterioration of vitamins. The answer is to chop, shred or grate the food immediately before cooking it.

Grilling [broiling] and frying Overcooking meat will destroy vitamin B1. And leaving the juices in the pan will cut down the iron content of the meal. So do keep grilled [broiled] and fried dishes rare, and use the juices for gravies or soups. Grilling [broiling] is also a good way of cooking fish.

Roasting and baking These are both good ways of cooking foods as long as you do not add too much extra fat. Wrap food in aluminium foil or transparent wrap so that it can cook in its own juices. And keep the delicious juices for gravies or stock.

Leftovers

Do not re-heat vegetables. Double cooking, plus possible keeping-warm time will destroy a very high proportion of the vitamin C content. Meat stews and broths can, however, be re-heated without much loss of nutrients because these are largely contained in the liquid surrounding the meat. Make sure they are thoroughly cooked however. Meat dishes that are re-heated should be brought to the boil quickly and boiled fast for 2-3 minutes, stirring constantly with a wooden spoon to avoid burning. Reduce the heat and simmer for 15 minutes. This ensures that any bacteria are destroyed.

The stockpot

Use leftover bones, poultry carcasses, fish pieces and vegetables to make nutritious stock—so useful as a base for many soups, sauces and stews. Brown meat bones in the oven, then put them in a large, heavy-bottomed pan with plenty of water. Add a few carrots, onions, turnips or other root vegetables, whole peppercorns and herbs. Bring to the boil and then simmer for 2-3 hours. This meat-based stock will keep for 3-4 days if you keep topping it up and boiling it every day —after that, discard it and start afresh. Fish and vegetable stocks can be made in the same way, without browning in the oven first. However, note that fish stocks, and stock which contains any green vegetables, should be used the same day, as they sour very quickly.

Salt and pepper

Use crystalline sea salt for cooking and at the table. Its main advantage used to be the iodine and other minerals which were usually removed from refined table salts. Nowadays, most table salts are iodized, so sea salt's pleasing texture and fresh taste are now its major recommendations. Use it with freshly ground black peppercorns for all your cooking needs.

re-think eating habits

There is no doubt that eating habits have deteriorated considerably over the last few years. It is this, rather than factory farming or food processing, which is primarily to blame for bad nutrition. After all, one helping of processed canned peas is hardly likely to hurt anyone. It is when those peas become the only green vegetable served at any meal that there is cause for concern. And, sadly, more and more people are depriving themselves of essential nutrients either through laziness, lack of interest or sheer ignorance.

Lack of time

Many people do not have a good, mixed diet. Instead, they subsist on hastily-prepared convenience foods, starchy snacks and confectionery. If they ate properly instead, then perhaps the cry for the preservation of minerals and vitamins in foods would be unnecessary. You can hardly blame manufacturers for producing the kind of goods that people want. Nor can you blame them for the fact that people are using items meant as useful additions to a diet as staple foods. (When the first frozen peas were marketed no one envisaged that a whole generation of children might grow up not knowing what a fresh pea tasted like!) But the manufacturers are, perhaps, encouraging the steady increase in bad eating habits with clever advertising.

Time rather than lack of money seems to be the main excuse for bad eating habits. Even an affluent family may be eating badly—particularly if the mother is too tired to shop daily for fresh produce. Here are some ideas to overcome this problem.

Shopping

If you work, shop once a week for main store-cupboard foods, weekend meat and bread. Use lunch-hours for buying fresh produce. Buy in small amounts that are easy to carry home—that way they will be fresher, too.

Cooking

Plan meals ahead—a week's menus at once if possible. To give yourself a proper rest have a mid-week roast and plan a cold picnic for the weekend. Prepare vegetables in advance if necessary and store in plastic bags in the refrigerator. They are just as quick to cook as canned or frozen vegetables. Use evenings or a free weekend to prepare a few nutritious snacks that the family can eat when you are not there to cook: open flans, wholemeal [wholewheat] scones, homemade soups, fresh fruit juices. Then, they will not be tempted in your absence to eat crisps [potato chips], sweets, sugary fruit drinks, etc.

Convenience foods

These are usually taken to mean the mass-produced, instant foods, but there are some superb natural foods which could just as well be called convenience foods. Milk is possibly the most convenient food of all. And fish is easy and quick to prepare when there is no time to cook a meat dish. Apples, bananas and oranges all travel well, need no special container and are fun to eat. Eggs come in their own extremely convenient packaging, and can be cooked in just three minutes. So there is no excuse for anyone to argue that they don't have the time to eat correctly.

Meal-times

Encourage the family to treat at least one meal of the day as a social occasion when they meet for a leisurely meal around a table. Avoid the tray meal

---

10 rules to help you break those bad eating habits

1. Eat a good breakfast every day, and make sure it supplies protein.
2. Never miss a meal.
3. Overcome a sweet tooth.
4. Pre-plan meals when possible.
5. Have nutritious snacks available for times when you cannot cook.
6. Be sure to buy fresh foods—fruit, vegetables, meat, fish—whenever possible.
7. Be aware of advertising pressure to buy confectionery and starchy foods, but do not succumb to it.
8. Make time to enjoy your food. Don't rush meals.
9. Plan your shopping list. Do not just dash around a supermarket selecting random items.
10. Remember that your example could influence others, especially children.

eaten in front of the television. If the family is in a rush, serve a really nutritious main course—a casserole, say—and fruit or cheese for dessert.

The dangers of refined sugar

In the West we now eat 20 times as much sugar as 200 years ago. The total yearly consumption is now around 45 pounds per head, a very large proportion of this being contained in manufactured foodstuffs—soft drinks, cakes, confectionery, ice-cream and baby foods. It could be argued that sugar supplies energy—and is therefore an important requirement in a healthy diet. However the word 'sugar' can be applied to various substances with similar, but not identical, properties. Some of the best known are glucose, fructose, maltose, lactose and sucrose. Sucrose is the substance which is found in refined table sugars and in sweetened foods. Glucose is found in fruits and vegetables, and is a key material in body metabolism. Sucrose, like glucose, converts rapidly into energy (i.e. converts into blood sugar), but it is usually stored as fat for future use because adequate supplies of sugar are found in fruits and some vegetables. And these foods have the advantage of providing vitamins and minerals as well as energy. Pure sugar provides energy but nothing else. And it is bad for your teeth and your figure too.

Fats—do you need them?

The dietary habit of always spreading butter or margarine on bread is peculiar to Western countries—where fat intake is usually above a healthy level, leading to overweight and possibly heart disease. The trouble is that the 'visible' fats—butter or margarine, fat on meat, lard, suet—make up only half the daily fat intake. The rest is 'invisible' fat supplied in the foods like eggs, cheese, milk, peanuts and some fish.

Fats are necessary as a concentrated source of energy. They build body fat to insulate against cold and give a protective, cushioning effect around some internal organs. And certain constituents of vegetable oils, the essential fatty acids, are necessary for correct growth and healthy skin.

What you must avoid is an excess of fat—vegetable or animal—which could lead to obesity problems. There is, too, a danger in the intake of too much saturated fat. This is found in animal fats and dairy products: meat, lard, butter and margarine.

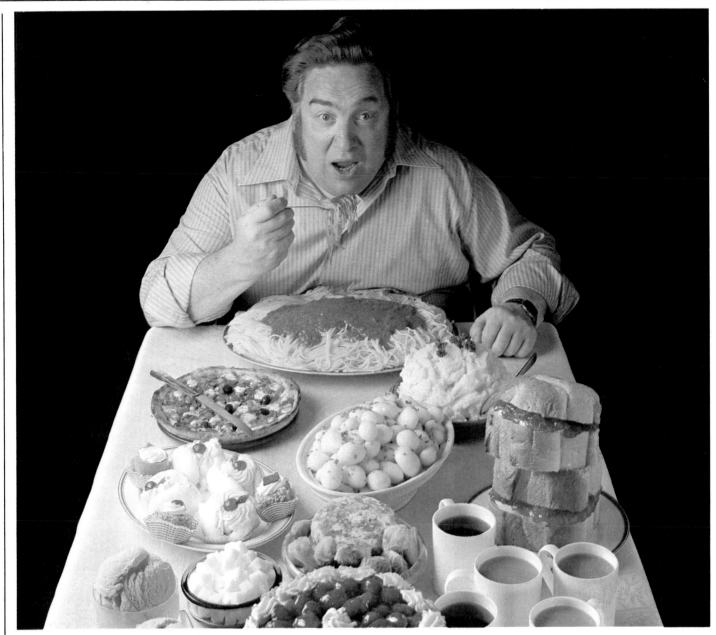

Vegetable oils—why they are better for you

Excessive quantities of cholesterol (hard fatty acids) and triglycerides (soft, buttery, fatty acids) can cause a build-up of fat in the blood and sometimes a blockage in the arteries. However, liquid, polyunsaturated fat is found in certain vegetable oils, sunflower seed and margarine made only from these oils. This fat does not produce a fatty acid build-up. The sensible way to include the best kinds of fat in your diet is to make sure that milk, eggs, lean meat, vegetables and vegetable oils figure strongly. If you have a family history of heart disease, or are in the 'danger' age-group of forty-plus, then it is wise to cut down on animal fats and use margarine made entirely from polyunsaturated fats. If you tend to be overweight, then avoid all the visible fats—your health will improve.

Liquid refreshment

Water-based drinks—tea, coffee and diluted soft drinks—are not as good for you as plain water. In fact, by mixing in popular beverage additions to water, you are simply adding your own toxins! Tannin (in tea) and caffeine (in coffee) are artificial stimulants which encourage acid secretion in the stomach which can, in turn, produce ulcers. They inhibit normal vitamin B metabolism and are definitely addictive! Scientists recently researching the stimulative effects of coffee on a group of students found that they experienced definite 'withdrawal' symptoms when supplies of the beverage were cut off. Headaches, dizziness and bad concentration ensued. Gradually, the symptoms passed and all subjects ultimately felt better without the artificial 'kick' of coffee.
Sweet drinks just load pure carbo-

hydrate into perfectly good water. They leave that sticky residue on the teeth which encourages dental caries, and their extra calories add inches.
The water-drinking habit is a good one. Add herbal teas and pure fruit and vegetable juices to your daily total fluid intake, and try to cut down consumption of tea and coffee.
The best alcoholic drinks in terms of food-value are beer, stout, mead (see p. 119) and red wine. Spirits supply little except calories! Beer and stout have the advantage of being rich in the 'B' vitamins (contained in the yeast with which they are made), plus a little protein, plenty of carbohydrate and minerals like potassium and chlorine. In fact, these are a good food choice, as long as the calories they supply are taken into account when the rest of the day's meals are planned. (For weight-watchers, champagne and dry red or white wine are the best choices.)

vitamin pills- do you need them?

If you eat properly then food supplements should be unnecessary. But who eats properly all the time? Even the most dedicated healthy foods addict must have the occasional glaring gaps in his or her nutritional programme:

the day when work pressures were too high to go out and buy an orange at lunchtime; the evening when friends came and there was no time for a cooked supper; the Sunday when the milkman forgot to call, and so it goes on.

It is, unfortunately, not really practical to give people a list of balanced, healthy foods and say piously; 'Stick to that every day and you'll never need to take a vitamin pill.' Most people, however well-intentioned, have at some time had a bout of bad eating that amounted to virtual malnutrition! One reason for such a lapse could be emotional. A sudden craving for sweet foods after a disagreement at home could mean the psychological association of sweet things with love. And psychologists say that people will often turn to foods they actually dislike in times of emotional crisis. So the 3-day chocolate and cake eating which hits a usually food-conscious teenager after an unhappy love-affair may be a subconscious reflex which is virtually

impossible to control. In such a situation it is no good saying that he or she must eat an orange and some meat to keep going. It is far better to produce a couple of vitamin pills and keep quiet until the crisis passes.

Then, too, built-in likes and dislikes can lead to diet deficiency. A pregnant woman who hates milk, cheese and yogurt will certainly suffer if her calcium intake is not bumped up with pills—even though she is a model of nutritional excellence when it comes to her weekly ration of liver and those daily green vegetables.

Men often suffer from vitamin C deficiency without even realizing it. They probably adore a huge steak with all its iron-rich juices and like a good cheese for dessert, but how many of them eat oranges or really enjoy green vegetables? If they seem to suffer from regular colds lack of vitamin C has probably a great deal to do with it. A daily pill could be a simpler, more effective, answer than persuading them to change their eating habits.

The trouble is that the water-soluble vitamins—C and B complex—must be taken daily. Five oranges on Monday will not, unfortunately, produce enough vitamin C to last until Friday. You need an orange every day, or a vitamin C pill. Check back with the chart of vitamins and minerals on pages 70-71, and remember that they are the minimum requirements. Now think back on what you ate yesterday. Did you really eat enough of everything? If not, a supplement might have been a good idea. This advice may seem to contradict what has been said previously. But people do need an escape clause. You may have firm intentions of eating well all the time, but it just is not possible to do so. Emotions, personal taste, or circumstances can, singly or together,. ruin the most carefully thought-out diet ideas

Do, however, be selective about supplements. Do not bother with all-embracing 'tonic' medicines or pills unless you are sure they are supplying sufficient quantities of the things which you lack. When you swallow a pill know what it contains and why you need it.

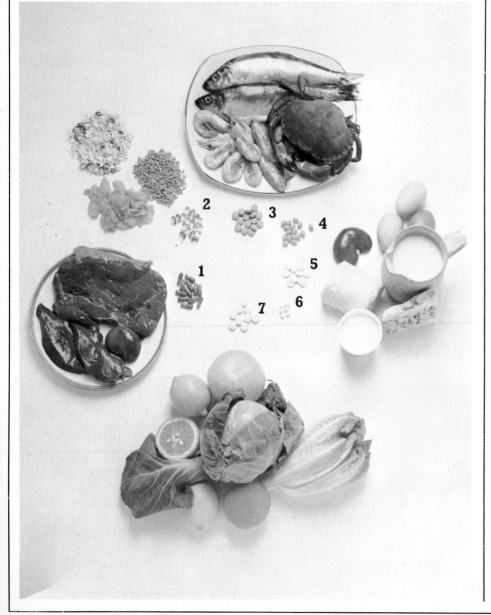

Check, and if you find you omit the food, take the pill. 1. Iron: in meat and eggs. 2. Vitamin E: in whole wheat and grain cereals. 3. Kelp: in sea foods. 4. Vitamin B complex: in dairy produce and kidneys. 5. Calcium: in milk, cheese and yogurt. 6. Vitamin A: in vegetables, offal and dairy products. 7. Vitamin C: in green vegetables and citrus fruit.

meat & poultry

Meat is one of the most vital sources of protein (about 27 per cent of the Western protein intake comes from it). Most families include at least one substantial meat dish in the day's meals, but all too often this takes the form of a grill or roast. Supermarkets are tending increasingly to eliminate the highly nutritious cheaper cuts of meat from their displays simply because people are not buying them. These cuts do require a little more preparation but as they help to vary the diet they are worth the effort. Badger your butcher or supermarket manager into providing these cheaper cuts and look for handy meat extras like beef bones to use for stocks, stews and soups. Gravies and sauces to accompany meat dishes are very important. They should be made with the meat juices in the pan as these contain much of the valuable iron content. Throw them away and you throw away nourishment. Roast meat in aluminium foil or a special closed roasting dish to preserve the flavour and juices, and always cover casseroles tightly. Buy meat near the time it is to be eaten—the same day, if possible. If you have to buy frozen meat, make sure it is thoroughly defrosted before use. Eating chicken which has not been properly thawed and thoroughly cooked can give you salmonella food poisoning.

Fairly bland-tasting meats like veal and the rather dull frozen chickens that most supermarkets sell can be considerably livened with a spice or herb-based marinade. The nutritional value of a battery chicken is the same as a free-range one but the taste certainly is not, so marinating may become an everyday cookery trick rather than a special-occasion one.

Offal [Variety Meats]

Liver, kidney and other offal [variety meats], like sweetbreads, brains, tongue and heart, are all highly nutritious. They contain vitamins A, the B complex and E (an important vitamin with few good sources), plus valuable minerals. Nutritionists recommend that liver should be included in the diet at least once a week especially for pregnant mothers and children. The trouble is that many people find offal unpalatable. Tough fried liver or boring stewed kidney is not likely to bring cries of joy from your family. But if you present these meats in their most attractive forms they are both tender and flavourful—and you'll be able to overcome any previous resistance.

Liver tossed with Onion and Caraway Seed Roast (recipes on next pages) are high in protein and easy to prepare.

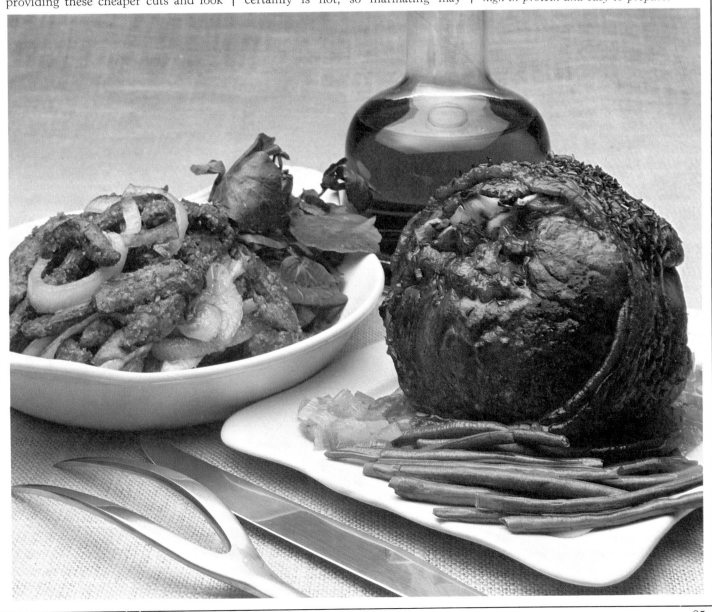

Caraway seed roast

This dish is particularly nutritious because of the added goodness from the beef bones. Serve with dumplings or potatoes baked in their jackets.
Preparation and cooking time:
1½ hours
SERVES 4-6

2 large onions, chopped
2 tablespoons caraway seeds
sea salt
2 lb. rib or sirloin of beef (boned)
2 oz. [4 tablespoons] bacon fat or dripping
2 tablespoons vinegar
freshly ground black pepper
2 lb. beef bones
water

Heat the oven to 425°F (Gas Mark 7, 220°C).
Mix 2 tablespoons of the chopped onion with 1 tablespoon of caraway seeds and a pinch of salt. Spread the meat with this mixture and roll and tie it with string. Put the rest of the chopped onion and the bacon fat into a roasting tin and cook it in the oven for 5 minutes.
Reduce the heat to 375°F (Gas Mark 5, 190°C).
Put the roll of meat into the tin, sprinkle it with the rest of the caraway seeds, the vinegar, and salt and pepper to taste. Arrange the beef bones around the meat and pour in water to come a quarter of the way up. Roast in the oven for an hour basting frequently.

Chicken barbecued with white wine

Although it is simple to prepare, this chicken dish tastes delicious. Try serving with a green salad for a summer lunch.
Preparation and cooking time:
45 minutes, plus 3 hours to marinate
SERVES 4

1 tablespoon chopped fresh rosemary
8 fl. oz. [1 cup] olive or corn oil
¼ bottle dry white wine
the juice of 1 lemon
2-2½ lb. roasting chicken
or 4 chicken pieces

Combine the rosemary, oil, wine and lemon. Cut the chicken into 4 pieces and marinate it in the rosemary mixture for 3 hours.

Remove the pieces from the marinade and grill them over a charcoal fire, or under a grill [broiler] for 45 minutes, brushing them frequently with the marinade.

Chicken with tarragon sauce

Chicken—always a favourite family lunch or dinner dish—is even better with this smooth herb sauce
Preparation and cooking time:
1 hour 45 minutes
SERVES 4-6

3-3½ lb. roasting chicken
vegetable oil
2-3 tablespoons chopped fresh tarragon or 1-2 tablespoons chopped dried tarragon
5 fl. oz. [⅝ cup] natural yogurt
sea salt
freshly ground black pepper
a squeeze of lemon juice

Heat the oven to 375°F (Gas Mark 5, 190°C).
Roast the chicken with a little vegetable oil for 1-1½ hours or until the juices run out clear when you pierce the bird with a skewer. Add the giblets to the pan when the fat begins to collect. As the chicken roasts, sprinkle well on all sides with tarragon. When cooked, place the chicken on an oven-proof dish and keep hot.
Pour the pan juices off into a small bowl, removing the giblets. Skim off most of the fat. Stir in the yogurt. Stand the bowl over a saucepan of hot water and heat gently. Season to taste with more tarragon, salt and pepper and a dash of lemon juice. (Prepared like this, the sauce should be hot but not boiling otherwise it may curdle. If it does it may be re-mixed in a blender and then returned to the bowl.)
Pour a little of the sauce over each helping of chicken and place the remainder in a separate bowl on the table.

Goulash with dumplings

This dish is a variation on the traditional goulash, and is delicious served with these dumplings.
Preparation and cooking time:
5½ hours
SERVES 2-4

2 oz. [4 tablespoons] dripping
1 lb. medium-sized onions, sliced
2 garlic cloves, crushed or sliced
1 lb. lean stewing beef cut into cubes
1 tablespoon paprika
salt
a pinch of marjoram
½ teaspoon caraway seeds
stock
1 lb. potatoes
For the dumplings:
8 oz. [2 cups] flour
salt
2 eggs
6 oz. [¾ cup] butter
water

Heat the oven to 300°F (Gas Mark 2, 150°C).
Melt the dripping in an ovenproof casserole and fry the onions and garlic in it for 5 minutes or until golden. Add the meat and brown it quickly on all sides. Add the paprika, salt, marjoram and caraway seeds. Add the stock so that it nearly covers the meat, and cook in the oven for 4-5 hours, adding the potatoes 30 minutes before the end of the cooking time.
Make the dumplings 1 hour before the end of the cooking time.
Sift together the flour and salt and put into a bowl. Make a well in the centre, break in the eggs and stir thoroughly. Melt half of the butter and add it to the mixture. Then add enough water to make a stiff dough.
Leave the dough in a cold place for 30 minutes.
With a warm spoon cut out teaspoon-fuls of the dough and cook these for 3 minutes in boiling water, then rinse them in cold water.
Just before serving melt the rest of the butter in a pan and heat the dumplings in it.

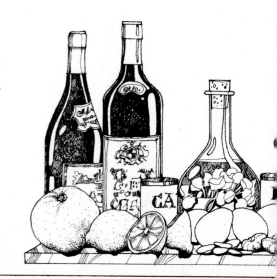

Hearts with apricot stuffing

This well-flavoured stuffing of fruit, nuts and wholemeal [wholewheat] crumbs turns an inexpensive meat into a very good supper dish.
Preparation and cooking time:
2 hours
S E R V E S 4

8 dried apricots
12 almonds, blanched and skinned
1 egg
2 tablespoons butter
1 oz. wholemeal [½ cup wholewheat] breadcrumbs
1 teaspoon sea salt
½ teaspoon freshly ground black pepper
1 orange
4 lambs' hearts, trimmed and cleaned
2 fl. oz. [¼ cup] chicken stock
1 tablespoon sherry
To garnish:
watercress

Heat the oven to 350°F (Gas Mark 4, 180°C).
Pour boiling water over the apricots and leave them to soak for 10 minutes.
Chop or mill the almonds. Beat the egg. Melt the butter in a small saucepan. Combine these with the breadcrumbs, season with salt and pepper. Drain the apricots, snip them into small pieces and add them to the mixture. Grate in 2 teaspoons of orange zest.
Pack the stuffing into hearts, secure with small larding skewers and place in an ovenproof dish. Pour the stock over, cover and bake in the oven for 1½ hours or until the hearts are tender.
Pour the juices from the dish into a small pan and boil briskly, to reduce. Squeeze the orange, add the orange juice and sherry to the pan and simmer for 5 minutes. Pour over the hearts and serve garnished with watercress.

Kidney and mushroom risotto

Unpolished rice retains the vitamins of the B complex. Cooking times are longer than for white rice, but the dish will have far more flavour.
Preparation and cooking time:
1 hour 10 minutes
S E R V E S 4

1 onion, peeled and chopped
2 tablespoons vegetable oil
2 oz. [¼ cup] butter
8 oz. [1⅓ cups] unpolished long-grain rice
1 pint [2½ cups] well-flavoured meat or vegetable stock
sea salt
freshly ground black pepper
8 lambs' kidneys, skinned and cored
4 oz. mushrooms
To garnish:
2 tablespoons chopped parsley

Melt half the butter with half the oil in a pan. Fry the onion gently in it for 5 minutes or until it is beginning to brown. Add the dry rice and continue to fry, stirring well, until the rice is golden.
Pour in three quarters of the stock. (A dash of wine or sherry could be added to the stock.) Season with salt and pepper, cover and simmer gently for 40-50 minutes. If it becomes too dry, add extra water or stock as necessary. When cooked, the rice should have absorbed all the liquid and be soft but not mushy.
Meanwhile prepare the kidneys and mushrooms. Slice the kidneys thickly and fry with the sliced mushrooms for 5 or 6 minutes over a fairly high heat in the remainder of the oil and butter. Then fork into the cooked rice, adding any pan juices.
Garnish with chopped parsley and serve.

Liver tossed with onion

Liver is made even more nutritious and tasty with this seasoning of kelp and wheat germ.
Preparation and cooking time:
20 minutes
S E R V E S 4

1½ lb. lamb or calf liver
1 large onion
3-4 tablespoons vegetable oil
1 tablespoon wholemeal [wholewheat] flour
1 tablespoon wheat germ
1 teaspoon kelp powder, or to taste
4 fl. oz. [½ cup] meat or vegetable stock
½ teaspoon yeast extract
To garnish:
watercress

Trim the liver and cut into thin strips.
Peel and slice the onion and fry in a little oil over medium heat for 5 minutes or until they begin to brown.
Mix together the flour, wheat germ and kelp. Toss the liver in the mixture. Then fry briskly in the pan with the onion for 4-5 minutes, turning occasionally, until just cooked. Transfer to a warm dish.
Add the stock and yeast extract to the pan, boil up for 2-3 minutes and pour over the liver.
Garnish with watercress and serve.

Liver with basil

The addition of basil gives a new flavour to the familiar liver and bacon.
Preparation and cooking time:
30 minutes
S E R V E S 4

1 oz. [2 tablespoons] butter
8 oz. bacon cut into strips
1 lb. lambs' liver, sliced
seasoned flour
2 tablespoons fresh chopped basil *or* 1 tablespoon dried basil
4 tablespoons red wine or stock

Melt the butter in a pan and fry the bacon. Remove it from the pan and keep warm.
Coat the liver slices in the seasoned flour and cook them in the butter for 5-7 minutes, turning all the time. Just before the liver is cooked add the basil and stock or red wine.
Arrange the liver on a plate with the bacon and pour over the pan juices.

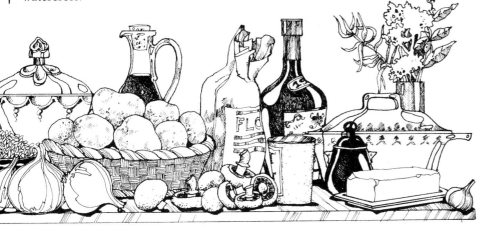

soups and casseroles-goodness preserved

One of the main points in favour of soups and casseroles is that you eat the vitamin-rich juices, instead of draining them away. And these dishes are an ideal way of using up vegetable water which you have conscientiously refrained from pouring down the sink.

The best bases for soups are these vegetable waters containing vitamin C, stock (see p.81) and pureéd vegetables like tomatoes, celery or carrots.

When selecting a lunch-time soup, remember that it should contain some protein if it is going to be the main course. So include grated cheese, beaten egg or lentils.

For slimmers, clear soups can be a good 'appetite-breaker' before the main course. They effectively take the edge off the appetite without adding too many extra calories to the meal total.

For invalids, soups are an excellent soothing introduction to solid food. But do make sure that they are nutritious as well—protein, vitamin C and iron can all be included in soup.

Once you have tasted a home-made soup the canned or powdered variety never tastes quite as good. But, when time is short, you can add your own 'extras' to patent soups: a little fresh sour cream and chopped parsley stirred into tinned lobster bisque, sherry and a few noodles added to consommé, chopped fresh tomatoes and grated cheese added to tinned tomato soup, or your own vegetable water with its valuable vitamin C residues added to a packet of dried mixed vegetable soup. These quick additions make a real difference to both flavour and goodness. Casserole cookery is another good way of blending and conserving valuable nutrients. Even the volatile vitamin C and iron (which so often escapes in meat juices) are safely contained in a tightly-closed casserole. Slow casserole cookery is a good way of using the less expensive cuts of meat and vegetables like carrots, potatoes and onions.

You can reheat casseroles but store them in the refrigerator until you want them. Never leave them in the oven.

Chilled summertime soup

This *gazpacho*-style cold soup is particularly delicious when served with sour cream.
Preparation and cooking time:
45 minutes
S E R V E S 4

1½ lb. ripe tomatoes
10 fl. oz. [1¼ cups] **chicken stock**
1 **large garlic clove**
2 **teaspoons sea salt**
2 oz. **wholemeal [1 cup wholewheat] breadcrumbs**
4 **tablespoons olive oil**
2 **tablespoons wine vinegar**
1 **large onion**
½ **cucumber**
1 **medium-sized green pepper**
¼ **teaspoon freshly ground black pepper**
a **pinch of ground cumin seed**
a **pinch of ground cardamom**
To serve:
sour cream
toasted or fried croûtons of wholemeal [wholewheat] bread

Scald the tomatoes in boiling water and skin them. Simmer gently in the stock for 10 minutes. Reduce to a purée in a blender or food mill, then rub through a coarse sieve to remove pips.
Peel the garlic and crush well with the salt using a knife blade. Mix the garlic, salt and breadcrumbs in a bowl and add the oil and vinegar, beating well. Combine with the sieved tomatoes, cover and chill until required.
Shortly before serving, peel the onion and cucumber and wash and de-seed the green pepper. Dice them all very finely and add half to the soup. Add pepper, cumin and cardamom to taste.
Serve from a bowl set in crushed ice with the remaining chopped vegetables, sour cream and toasted or fried croûtons of wholemeal [wholewheat] bread in separate bowls.

Clear vegetable soup with cheese and yogurt

This recipe could be served alone, with a simple chopped parsley garnish or with the yogurt and cheese garnish suggested for extra protein.
Preparation and cooking time:
45 minutes
S E R V E S 6

8 oz. **mushrooms**
3 **tablespoons butter**
2 **carrots**
1 **onion**
½ **celery stalk**
4 oz. **green beans**
1½ pints [3¾ cups] **stock or water**
sea salt
freshly ground black pepper
6 **tablespoons natural yogurt**
4 **tablespoons grated Parmesan cheese**

Wash the mushrooms and slice thinly. Melt 1 tablespoon of butter in a saucepan, add the sliced mushrooms and cook for 2 minutes.
Clean the rest of the vegetables and cut them into thin slices. Cook in a little of the stock or water for 5 minutes. Add the rest of the stock or water, bring to the boil and simmer for about 30 minutes. Season, add the mushrooms and simmer for a further 5 minutes.
Just before serving, stir a tablespoon of yogurt into each soup portion, and sprinkle with grated Parmesan cheese.

Onion soup

This healthy, uncomplicated onion soup is delicately flavoured with herbs.
Preparation and cooking time:
45 minutes
S E R V E S 4-6

6 medium-sized onions
1 garlic clove
2 oz. [4 tablespoons] butter
1 pint [2½ cups] water, boiling
1½ pints [3¾ cups] stock, heated
1 bouquet garni
freshly ground black pepper
sea salt
1 egg, beaten
3 drops wine vinegar

Peel and slice the onions and chop
the garlic. Melt the butter in a pan
and add the onions and garlic. Cook
them over medium heat for 5 minutes
or until soft.
Pour on the boiling water, stir well,
and add the stock. Put in the bouquet
garni, season, and simmer for 30
minutes.
Remove the pan from the heat and take
out the bouquet garni. Stir in the
beaten egg and the vinegar and,
serve at once.

Pork casserole

This is a satisfying dish, subtly
flavoured with thyme.
Preparation and cooking time:
1½ hours
SERVES 3-4

1 lb. lean pork
3 medium-sized onions
2 tablespoons butter
1 tablespoon flour
15 fl. oz. [2 cups] stock
2 celery stalks
½ teaspoon chopped, fresh thyme
    or ¼ teaspoon dried thyme
sea salt
freshly ground black pepper

Heat the oven to 350°F (Gas Mark 4,
180°C).
Cut the meat into cubes and peel and
chop the onions.
Melt the butter in an ovenproof
casserole and sauté the pork and
onions in it until browned. Remove
from the heat and stir in the flour.
Pour the stock over and simmer.
Meanwhile, clean and chop the
celery and then add it to the casserole
with the thyme, and salt and pepper
to taste. Cover and bake in the oven
for about 1 hour, or until the meat
is tender.

*To give soups and casseroles a new look
try using different combinations of
flavours or unusual vegetables—celery
with chicken say, or root vegetables
with cheap cuts of meat.*

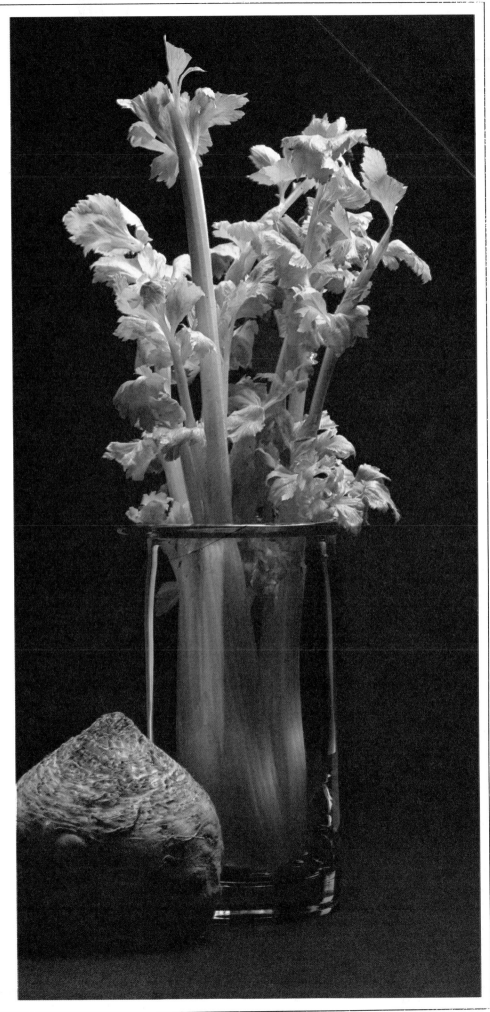

fish

Fish is an excellent source of protein and of vitamin B (niacin). Oily fish like herring, mackerel and salmon are also good sources of vitamins A and D. Iodine comes from salt-water fish and shellfish and there is simply no other common source of it.

All this means that fish can, and should, play an important part in a well-balanced diet. Fresh fish is best for flavour, but frozen or canned fish (particularly canned oily fish) are also good buys. When shopping for fresh fish look for firm flesh, sparkling silvery scales, red gills, bright eyes and a sweet fresh smell. (Fresh fish does not smell offensive.)

Cook fish quickly. Never boil it for too long. Either poach it lightly or, for the best results, grill [broil], fry or bake in foil. Never re-heat a fish dish; eat it immediately after cooking.

The roe is the part of the fish richest in the B vitamins. It can be delicious grilled and served alone as a supper dish. Use the fish bones and heads to make fish stock. This is useful as a basis for soups and other fish dishes. Try the recipes below and experiment with your own ideas. Fish can be just as versatile as meat and it has the added advantage of being quick to cook. It generally makes a lighter dish, too, and so is often more suitable for a quick lunch than a heavy meat dish would be.

Baked cod

This is an interesting way of serving cod, and it is much better for you than frying it in batter.
Preparation and cooking time:
1 hour
S E R V E S 4-6

2 lb. cod
2 pints [5 cups] **fish stock** *or*
    water
1 **bouquet garni**
sea salt
freshly ground black pepper
3 oz. wholemeal [1½ cups
    wholewheat] **breadcrumbs**
3 tablespoons **flour**
2 oz. [4 tablespoons] **butter**
1 pint freshly-shelled (1 lb. frozen)
    shrimps

1 tablespoon **anchovy essence**
To garnish:
1 **lemon, sliced**
parsley

Heat the oven to 350°F (Gas Mark 4, 180°C).
Wash and dry the fish, put it in a baking tin and add the stock, the bouquet garni, salt and pepper. Mix together the breadcrumbs and flour, cover the fish with this mixture and dot with the butter.
Bake in a moderate oven, basting frequently, for about 30 minutes.
Take 4 tablespoons of the liquid out of the dish, pour it over the shrimps and mix in the anchovy essence. Pour this shrimp mixture over the fish, return it to the oven and bake for a further 7 minutes.
Garnish with lemon slices and parsley.
(For the bouquet garni use a traditional one consisting of 4 parsley sprigs, 1 thyme spray and 1 bay leaf tied together. Alternatively, try bay, fennel and lemon rind or lemon balm.)

Baked stuffed mackerel

Mackerel is a tasty and inexpensive fish, and is particularly good with this piquant stuffing.
Preparation and cooking time:
45 minutes
S E R V E S 4

4 good-sized **mackerel, cleaned and
    boned**
2 oz. [½ cup] **oatmeal**
4 oz. [½ cup] **butter**
1 small **onion**
¼ teaspoon **freshly ground black
    pepper**
½ teaspoon **ground bay leaves**
¼ teaspoon **kelp powder**
sea salt
1 tablespoon **wheat germ**

Heat the oven to 375°F (Gas Mark 5, 190°C).
Wash the fish well and dry on kitchen paper. Mix the oatmeal and half the butter with a fork. Chop the onion finely and combine it with the oatmeal and butter. Season with the pepper, ground bay leaves and kelp, adding a little more if preferred, and a grinding of sea salt to taste.
Blend together well.
Pack this stuffing into the fish, lay them on a large piece of buttered

aluminium foil. Dot with the rest of the butter and gather the foil loosely together over the top of the fish.
Bake for 15-20 minutes or until the fish is cooked through.
Open the foil, sprinkle the fish with wheat germ and crisp under the grill [broiler] before serving.

Creamy shrimp scallops

This delicious hot first course looks very attractive served in scallop shells.
Preparation and cooking time:
40 minutes
S E R V E S 4

1 **shallot, chopped finely**
1 tablespoon **butter**
5 fl. oz. [⅝ cup] **natural yogurt**
2 **egg yolks**
8 oz. cooked **shrimps, shelled**
2 teaspoons chopped **parsley**
sea salt
freshly ground black pepper
1 tablespoon grated **Parmesan
    cheese**

Heat the oven to 350°F (Gas Mark 4, 180°C).
Cook the chopped shallot in the butter until soft.
Beat the yogurt and egg yolks together. Stir in the shrimps, the softened shallot and parsley. Season to taste.
Pour into scallop shells or greased ramekin dishes and sprinkle with Parmesan cheese. Bake for 25 minutes until set and golden.

Fish fillets, Spanish style

White fish combines well with the rich flavours of green peppers, mushrooms and tomatoes.
Preparation and cooking time:
45 minutes
S E R V E S 4

1½ lb. **cod fillet**
1 medium-sized **onion**
1 **garlic clove**
1 **celery stalk**
½ medium-sized **green pepper**
4 oz. **mushrooms**
8 oz. **tomatoes**
2 tablespoons **butter**
1 tablespoon **corn oil**
3 fl. oz. [⅜ cup] **water**
1 tablespoon **tomato purée**

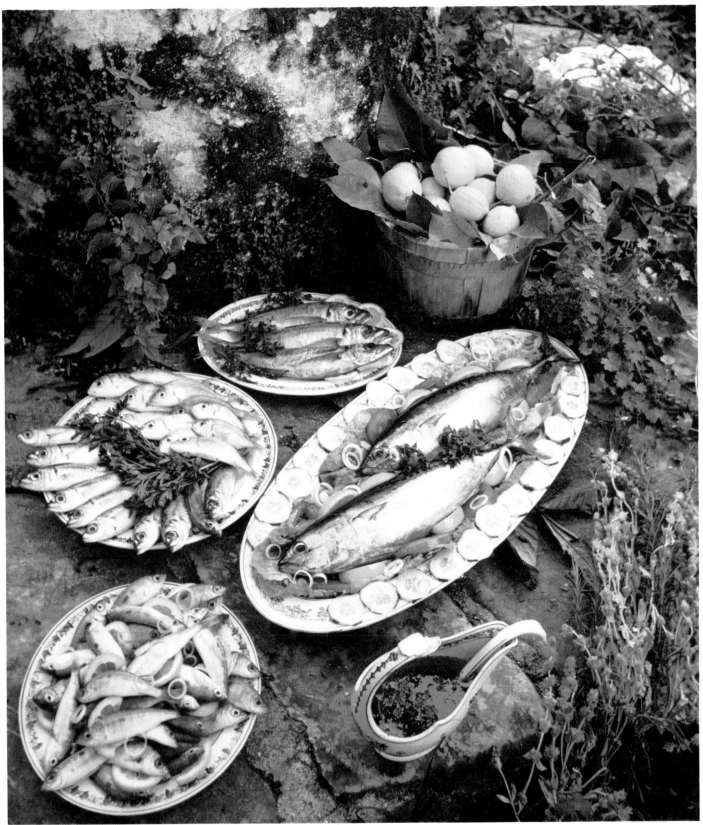

1 tablespoon white wine
sea salt
freshly ground black pepper
Worcestershire sauce
To garnish:
chopped parsley

Poach the fish gently in lightly salted water for 15-20 minutes or until it is cooked through but still firm. Then drain and keep hot.

Meanwhile, peel and chop the onion, crush the garlic, wash and finely chop the celery and de-seed and chop the green pepper. Wash, dry and chop the mushrooms, skin and chop the tomatoes.
Melt the butter and oil in a heavy pan and fry onion and garlic gently for a few minutes. Add the rest of the vegetables, the water, tomato purée and wine. Simmer for about 20

Quick to cook, flavourful and extremely versatile, fish provides both protein and vitamins.

minutes or until soft and thick, adding a little more water if it reduces too much.
Season the sauce to taste with salt, pepper and Worcestershire sauce. Pour the sauce over the fish. Garnish with plenty of chopped parsley and serve.

cheese

Cheese is one of the most versatile and nourishing foods available. It really does contribute a great deal to a balanced diet. It is full of protein (weight for weight, Cheddar cheese supplies marginally more than best fillet steak), and contains vitamins A, B, B2, and E. The immense variety of dishes, sauces and snacks you can prepare with just a good piece of cheese as a starting point makes it one of the best possible buys. Cheddar or one of the other hard cheeses is best for cooking, and it can be slightly stale. (For grating, the harder it is the better.) For salads, on the other hand, the cheese should be firm and fresh. Creamy fresh-tasting cottage cheese is particularly good in salads. Processed cheese is useful as a store-cupboard standby, but is unsuitable for cooking because it contains extra water and additives. Cheese should be stored in a cool place, covered loosely. It will go hard quickly if it is entirely exposed to air. And if it is tightly covered it is likely to mould. Although cheese often requires months, or years, to ripen to full maturity, once ripe it does deteriorate rapidly. So buy it in fairly small quantities—enough to last just a few days. There are so many uses for cheese that there should be no problem in finishing it off quickly. Below are some quick ideas, but try the recipes, too.

Dips
Make a cold cheese dip with cream cheese or cottage cheese and sour cream combined with a dash of prepared mustard. Serve with raw carrots or other crisp raw vegetables.

Dressing and garnishes
Grated cheese is a good garnish for soups and vegetables. (Brown it under the grill [broiler] if you like.) Crumbled Roquefort or Danish blue cheese mixed with natural yogurt makes a good dressing to serve with salads.

Hot snacks
Add a couple of quick cheese bakes to your repertoire. Slices of ham rolled around cooked chicory, topped with a cheesy sauce and baked in the oven taste delicious. So do green peppers filled with a minced [ground] beef or nut-based stuffing, topped with grated cheese and baked.

Cottage cheese and mushroom quiche

This lunch or supper dish uses eggs and the added protein of cottage cheese. It may be served either with vegetables or a green salad.
Preparation and cooking time:
1½ hours
SERVES 4-6

6 oz. [1½ cups] flour
a pinch of sea salt
3 oz. [⅜ cup] margarine
water
For the filling:
1 tablespoon chopped onion
2 tablespoons vegetable oil
6-8 mushrooms, sliced
3 eggs
8 oz. cottage cheese
2 oz. cooked ham *or* boiled bacon, chopped
2 tablespoons chopped fresh tarragon
1 teaspoon sea salt
a pinch of freshly ground black pepper

Heat the oven to 425°F (Gas Mark 7, 220°C).
Sift together the flour and salt and rub in the margarine. Add just enough water to make a firm dough. Roll out and use it to line a greased 8-inch pie plate.
Fry the onion gently in a little oil until soft but not brown. Add mushrooms and cook until they begin to soften.
Beat the eggs and mix well with the cottage cheese. Add the onion and mushroom with the ham or bacon, tarragon and seasoning.
Pour mixture into the prepared pastry case and bake for 15 minutes. Lower the heat to 350°F (Gas Mark 4, 180°C) and bake for a further 40 to 50 minutes, or until the filling has risen and is firm to the touch.

Cottage cheese and smoked fish cocottes
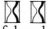

The fish and cottage cheese flavours complement each other particularly well in this dish.
Preparation and cooking time:
1½ hours
SERVES 4

8 oz. smoked haddock or kipper fillets, fresh or frozen

8 oz. cottage cheese
1 medium-sized onion, chopped and lightly cooked in butter
4 oz. mushrooms, chopped
2 eggs
the juice of 1 lemon
sea salt
freshly ground black pepper
To garnish:
lemon twists
parsley sprigs

Heat the oven to 375°F (Gas Mark 5, 190°C).
Poach smoked fish in a little milk. Skin and flake the fish and mix with the cottage cheese, onion and mushrooms. Beat the eggs and add to mixture. Add lemon juice and season to taste.
Grease 4 cocotte or ramekin dishes and divide the mixture between them. Stand in a baking tin of warm water and bake in the oven for 40 minutes or until set.
Garnish with lemon twists and sprigs of parsley.

Cottage cheese lunch platter

This is a good light lunch dish, which could also be served as a first course. Other fresh herbs such as basil and tarragon may be used, but they should always be added cautiously, tasting as you go.
Preparation time:
45 minutes
SERVES 4

1 medium-sized cucumber
4 large tomatoes
1 small lettuce
8 oz. cottage cheese
1 tablespoon chopped fresh chives
4 spikes fresh rosemary, chopped
1 teaspoon chopped thyme
1 teaspoon chopped lemon balm
½ teaspoon dried caraway seeds
2 tablespoons sour cream
1 teaspoon sea salt
¼ teaspoon freshly ground black pepper
To garnish:
sprigs of parsley

Peel the cucumber, cut into 8 pieces and remove seeds. Sprinkle well with salt and leave for 30 minutes.
Wash the tomatoes, cut a slice from the tops and scoop out the seeds. Save the slices for garnish.

Wash the lettuce, dry and wrap in a cloth. Crisp in the refrigerator until required.

Turn the cottage cheese into a bowl and mix in the chopped herbs, sour cream and seasonings. Taste and add more salt and pepper if required.

Drain the moisture from the cucumber pieces, and arrange the lettuce leaves on a serving platter. Pack the herby cottage cheese filling into the tomatoes and cucumber pieces and arrange them on the lettuce.

Garnish with sprigs of parsley and slivers from tomato tops.

Pizza with cheese and olives

⧖ ⧖

This pizza, based on an easy yeast dough, makes a complete meal if you serve it with a crisp salad. Alternatively, serve it in small portions as a first course.
Preparation and cooking time:
1 hour 50 minutes
SERVES 6-8

For the pizza base:
½ teaspoon sugar
3 tablespoons tepid water (110°F, 43°C)
½ tablespoon dried yeast
8 oz. wholemeal [2 cups wholewheat] flour
1 teaspoon sea salt
2 eggs
2 oz. [¼ cup] soft butter
For the topping:
1 lb. ripe tomatoes
1 medium-sized onion
1 small garlic clove
1 tablespoon cooking oil
½ teaspoon sea salt
¼ teaspoon black pepper
3 oz. sharp cheese
1 teaspoon chopped fresh marjoram
 or ½ **teaspoon dried marjoram**
1 teaspoon chopped fresh thyme
 or ½ **teaspoon dried thyme**
½ **teaspoon chopped fresh rosemary**
 or ¼ **teaspoon dried rosemary**
12 black olives
1 tablespoon capers (optional)

Stir the sugar into the water, sprinkle the yeast on top and leave for 10 minutes.

Mix the flour and salt together in a warm bowl. Beat the eggs into the yeast liquid and add to the flour. Work in the butter.

Cover the bowl with a clean cloth and set it in a warm, draught-free place. Leave it for 45 minutes, or until the dough has risen and doubled in bulk.

Meanwhile, make the topping. Scald the tomatoes in boiling water, skin and chop roughly. Peel and chop the onion. Skin and crush the garlic. Fry the onion and garlic gently in the oil until soft and translucent, then add the tomatoes. Cook to a soft purée, then turn up the heat to reduce. Turn into a bowl to cool and season with salt and pepper.

Heat the oven to 400°F (Gas Mark 6, 200°C).

Flour a baking sheet. Place the risen

Use cottage cheese, a cheap source of protein, either cold in a lunch platter or hot in a quiche.

dough on it and pat into a 9-inch circle. Spread the tomato mixture on top, leaving a half-inch border.

Grate the cheese over the top, sprinkle with the herbs and garnish with the olives and capers.

Leave the pizza for 15 minutes in a warm place to allow the dough to rise again, then bake for 20-25 minutes until browned and cooked through.

yogurt

Yogurt—what it is, and what it can do for you

'Yogurt' is in fact the Bulgarian and Turkish name for fermented milk—but it has many other names. In India it is called *dahi*; in the Balkans, *tarho*; in the Eastern Carpathians, *huslanka*; in Southern Russia and the Caucasus, *kefir* or *kuban*; in Egypt and most of Asia Minor, *leben* or *laban*, in Siberia and Central Asia, *koumiss*.

Yogurt has become popular in Western countries only during recent years, but it has for many centuries been part of the everyday diet of people in Eastern Europe, the Middle and Far East and Africa. Milk—from cows, sheep or goats—was one of the basic foods of many tribes and civilizations and as it does not stay fresh for very long, people experimented to find a way to make sour milk palatable. Fermentation, perhaps using a piece of decaying vegetable or animal matter to trigger off the process, was found to be the answer to the problem. The flavour and consistency of the finished yogurt varied from country to country and tribe to tribe depending on the method and length of fermentation, the type of milk and the kind of feeding stuff used for the animals.

The first scientific investigations into yogurt were made by Metchnikoff in 1907 at the Pasteur Institute in Paris. He was attracted by the idea that people living in Bulgarian villages ate vast quantities of sour milk and were supposed to live for a very long time —100 years or more. He studied the substance, and isolated a strong lactic acid-producing organism. This he named 'long-life bacillus' and it is used in the making of today's yogurt.

How yogurt is made

Yogurt contains all the food value of milk, but it has most of the fat removed and extra protein and vitamins added. Yogurt is commercially prepared from fresh, high-quality milk and is extremely good for you, but homemade yogurt is infinitely preferable. This is not because it is any more nutritious —in fact, it isn't—but it has a flavour and texture that commercially prepared yogurt never has.

Never freeze yogurt, store it in a refrigerator or cold larder and it will keep for two weeks or more quite safely. If it is kept in a warm room its acid content increases rapidly and this gives the yogurt a 'sharper' taste which many people find unpleasant.

Food value

Yogurt is an important source of protein. (See chart p.68). It also has the advantage of being highly digestible—about three times as digestible as milk —which makes it a good food for invalids or anyone feeling fragile.

For slimmers, there is also the advantage of protein without excessive calories. (5 ounces of low-fat unsweetened yogurt would supply about 75 calories whereas two slices of lean beef supply 150 calories.)

Versatility

Yogurt is not only nutritious; it is also, for the imaginative and health-conscious cook, marvellously versatile. It is included in recipes coming from many countries. In India yogurt is eaten with meat and vegetable curries, with sugar, honey, fruit and molasses. In Russia it is added to soups and stews. In Bulgaria and Turkey it is an important ingredient in many delicious dishes.

The consistency and bland flavour of yogurt bring out and subtly add to many other food flavours. It has the versatility of cream, without the fat content.

Yogurt machines

The main problem in making your own yogurt is to keep the milk warm for the 10-16 hours while fermentation takes place. One good way to overcome this difficulty is to use an electric yogurt-making machine with a thermostatically controlled fermentation chamber. These all come with specific instructions but the basic method is simply to place one tablespoon of shop-bought yogurt in the chamber, top up with milk, switch on and leave overnight.

Vitamins

All commercial yogurts supply valuable quantities of the 'B' vitamins, but quantities of vitamins A and D vary from brand to brand. (One very popular brand supplies 603 International Units of vitamin A per 100 grams and 83.3 International Units of vitamin D per 100 grams.)

Blackberry cooler

This is a light and digestible yogurt drink to make when it is too hot to eat a full meal.
Preparation and cooking time:
10 minutes, plus chilling time
S E R V E S 4

8 oz. blackberries
10 fl. oz. [1¼ cups] natural yogurt
2 egg yolks
2 tablespoons clear honey, or to taste

Stew the blackberries with just enough water to prevent them sticking to the pan, for 4 or 5 minutes, pressing down with a spoon to extract the juice. Rub them through a fine sieve to remove pips. Chill the purée until required.
Combine blackberry purée, yogurt, egg yolks and honey in a blender and blend at full speed for 2 minutes. Then serve.

Homemade natural yogurt

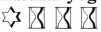

Making yogurt at home is quite simple, but it often has a thin consistency. This method gives a closer curd which is preferable for most desserts.
Preparation time:
30 minutes, plus 12 hours to incubate the yogurt
M A K E S 1 pint [2½ cups]

1 pint [2½ cups] milk
3 tablespoons dried skimmed milk powder (not instant granules)
1 tablespoon commercial live yogurt

Bring the milk to the boil, lower heat and simmer for 5 minutes. Remove to a bowl and cool to blood heat. (If the milk is too warm, the yogurt will separate.) The bowl may be placed in iced water to speed up cooling.
Sprinkle the skimmed milk powder on to the milk and mix it in with a fork. Stir in the live yogurt.
Turn the mixture into a wide-mouthed vacuum jar which has been rinsed out with warm water, close and leave for 12 hours or overnight. Turn out and refrigerate until needed.

Homemade Yogurt (top) is used to make a Yogurt and Orange Whip (below).

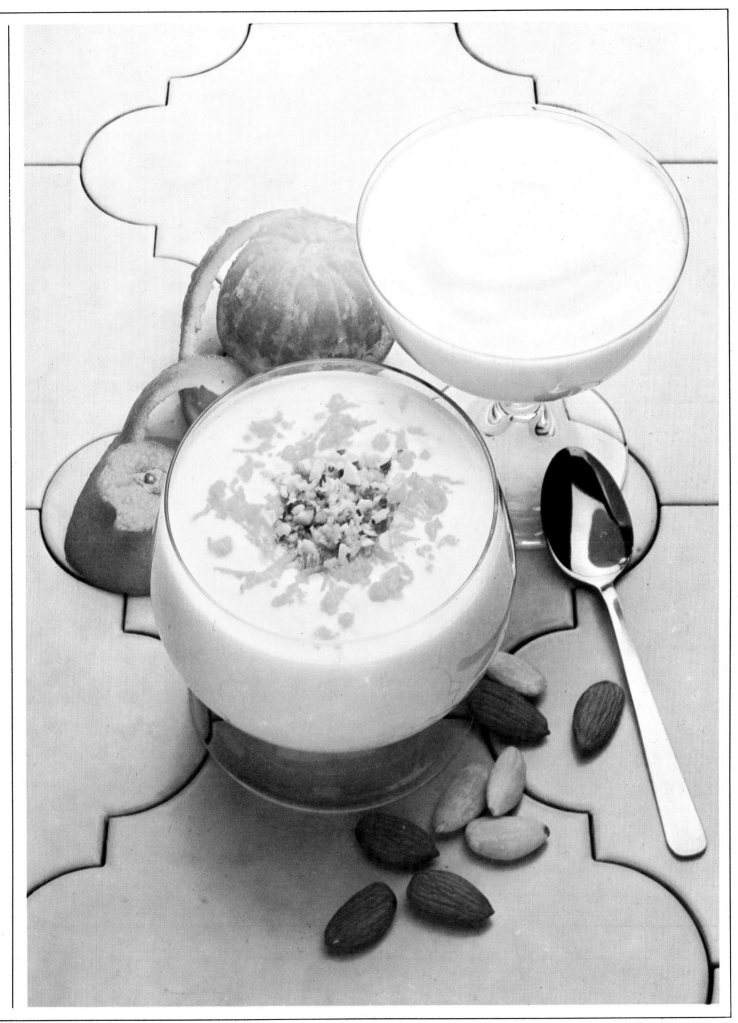

Lemon consommé with yogurt

This is a light, refreshing cold soup with a sharp, tangy taste.
Preparation and cooking time:
10 minutes, plus setting time
S E R V E S 4

16 fl. oz. [2 cups] **consommé** (canned)
2 teaspoonfuls dry sherry
the juice and grated zest of ½ lemon
10 fl. oz. [1¼ cups] **natural yogurt**
3 sprigs fresh or 2 sprigs dried
   tarragon, if available

Warm together the consommé, sherry and lemon juice. Pour into individual soup bowls and chill. *Combine* the grated lemon zest, yogurt and tarragon. When the consommé has set, and just before serving, remove the sprigs of tarragon from yogurt, then spoon it on to consommé.

Oriental dressing

This goes well with any salad which combines fruit and vegetables. It is also good served with cold meats.
Preparation time:
5 minutes, plus chilling time
M A K E S 5 fluid ounces

5 fl. oz. [⅝ cup] **natural yogurt**
1 teaspoon **curry powder**
¼ teaspoon finely grated **lemon zest**
2 teaspoons **lemon juice**
½ teaspoon chopped **mixed herbs**
¼ teaspoon **sea salt**

Combine all the ingredients and chill well before serving.

Piquant dressing

This has a tangy flavour which is marvellous with a salad.
Preparation time: *5 minutes*
M A K E S 5 fluid ounces

5 fl. oz. [⅝ cup] **natural yogurt**
1 tablespoon chopped **chives**
¼ teaspoon dry mustard
¼ teaspoon garlic salt
1 teaspoon **lemon juice**
sea salt
freshly ground black pepper

Combine all the ingredients and serve immediately.

Watercress dressing

Watercress has a strong, pungent flavour and is rich in iron and vitamin E. This dressing is good with roast meats, especially beef.
Preparation time:
5 minutes
M A K E S 5 fluid ounces

a small bunch **watercress**
5 fl. oz. [⅝ cup] **natural yogurt**
½ teaspoon **lemon juice**
sea salt
freshly ground black pepper

Remove the coarse stalks from the watercress. Chop the rest finely. Mix in the yogurt and lemon juice and season to taste.

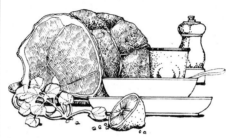

Yogurt and orange whip

This refreshing and tangy summer dessert can be made with any fruit. But you do need a blender to make it successfully.
Preparation time:
15 minutes, plus 2 hours chilling time
S E R V E S 4

8 medium-sized **oranges**
2 tablespoons **honey**
1 pint [2½ cups] **yogurt**
4 tablespoons chopped **walnuts,
   almonds or hazelnuts**

Peel the oranges, removing as much of the white pith as possible. Reserve about 2 teaspoons of the orange rind and chop it finely. Set aside.
Chop the orange flesh into small pieces with a serrated-edge knife, and place them in a blender. Add the honey and yogurt and blend at high speed for about 20 seconds, or until the ingredients are well combined.
Pour the orange mixture into four individual glass serving dishes. Place them in the refrigerator and chill for at least 2 hours.
Just before serving, sprinkle the tops with the nuts and reserved orange rind.

vegetables

Vegetables deserve to be cooked with as much care and attention as meat. They can stand alone very successfully too. The European idea of serving the vegetable course separately from the meat is a good one. After a cooked meat dish, a clean-tasting dish of short-cooked green vegetables or a vegetable salad provides a change of texture and some work for digestive juices. (And it adds roughage to the meal, especially if the vegetables are crunchy and chewy.)
Food values in vegetables vary according to the way they are stored before cooking, and how you cook them. Vitamin C is volatile. It dissolves in water and evaporates with moisture if the vegetables are exposed to the air. Vitamin A, which is found in things like carrots, loses potency through heat. So cook vegetables quickly in very little water, and serve them still crunchy.
There are three substantial vegetable dishes in this section: a curry, a casserole and a couscous. There is also a bean salad. And this raises the subject of which vegetables are suitable for salads. Lettuce, tomatoes and cucumbers may be the favourites but shredded raw cabbage, cold cooked potatoes, spinach leaves, grated carrot, grated turnip and cauliflower are just as suitable. (The dressing given for the Bean Salad is also delicious used with all the vegetables above.)

Aubergine [Eggplant] casserole

The aubergine [eggplant] is an exotic vegetable that is also very adaptable. This recipe is Middle Eastern in origin but its marvellous flavour will appeal to everyone. Serve the casserole hot or cold.
Preparation and cooking time:
2¼ hours
S E R V E S 4

10 oz. dried **chick-peas, soaked
   overnight and drained** or 14 oz.
   canned **chick-peas, drained**
1½ pints [3¾ cups] **water**
2 medium-sized **aubergines
   [eggplants]**
1½ teaspoons **sea salt**

7 fl. oz. [⅞ cup] olive oil
4 small courgettes [zucchini]
washed, trimmed and sliced into
¼-inch slices
2 medium-sized onions, sliced
2 garlic cloves, crushed
8 oz. canned peeled tomatoes,
drained and chopped with liquid
reserved
½ teaspoon cayenne pepper
1 teaspoon ground cumin

If you are using dried chick-peas,
put them into a large saucepan and
pour in the water. Place the pan
over moderately high heat and bring
the water to the boil. Reduce the
heat to low, partially cover the pan
and cook for 45 minutes, or until the
peas are just tender. Remove the pan
from the heat and drain the chick-
peas in a colander. Set aside. (If
you are using canned chick-peas, the
above step can be omitted.)
Meanwhile, peel the aubergines
[eggplants] and dice the flesh.
Place the pieces in a colander and
sprinkle them with 1 teaspoon of
the salt. Leave them for 30 minutes,
then drain on kitchen paper towels.
Heat 4 fluid ounces [½ cup] of the
oil in a large frying pan over
moderate heat. When the oil is hot,
add the chopped aubergine [eggplant]
and cook, stirring occasionally, for
10 minutes, or until the pieces are
evenly browned on all sides.
Transfer the aubergine [eggplant]
and any cooking liquid to a large
mixing bowl.
Heat the oven to 350°F (Gas Mark 4,
180°C).
Heat the remaining oil in the frying
pan, over moderate heat. When the
oil is hot, add the courgette
[zucchini] slices to the pan. Cook
them, stirring occasionally, for 8 to
10 minutes, or until they are evenly
browned. With a slotted spoon,
transfer the courgette [zucchini]
slices to the mixing bowl with the
aubergines [eggplants]. Set aside.
Add the onions and garlic to the pan
and cook them, stirring occasionally,
for 5-7 minutes, or until the
onions are soft and translucent but
not brown. Add the tomatoes, the
remaining salt, the cayenne and cumin
to the pan and stir well to mix.
Cook the tomato mixture for 3
minutes, then remove the pan from
the heat and stir the mixture into the
aubergine [eggplant] mixture. Stir in
the chick-peas and the reserved
tomato juice.
Transfer the mixture to a deep
ovenproof casserole. Place it

in the centre of the oven and bake
for 1 hour, or until all of the
vegetables are tender. Serve at once.
(If you want to serve the casserole
cold, allow it to cool to room
temperature, then place it in the
refrigerator to chill for at least
2 hours.)

Bean salad

Serve this with cold meat or as part
of a summer buffet meal.
Preparation and cooking time:
30 minutes
SERVES 2-4

1 lb. green beans
2 tablespoons olive *or* sunflower
oil
the juice of 1 lemon
1 medium-sized onion
1 clove garlic (optional)
1 teaspoon chopped parsley
1 teaspoon chopped savory
sea salt
freshly ground black pepper
a few lettuce leaves
To garnish:
1 egg, hard-boiled and chopped

Cook the beans in a little boiling
salted water until tender, drain and
cool.
Mix the oil and lemon juice. Slice the
onion finely and slice or crush
garlic and mix into the dressing,
adding the herbs and seasoning. Pour
dressing over the beans.
Pile the beans on to the lettuce
leaves and serve garnished with the
egg.

Curry creole

This spicy yet refreshing mixture
of fruit and vegetables makes a
delightful summer supper dish.
Serve it with boiled rice and a
tossed green salad.
Preparation and cooking time:
1 hour
SERVES 4

4 oz. [½ cup] butter or margarine
2 medium-sized onions, thinly
sliced
1 garlic clove, crushed
1 green chilli, de-seeded and
chopped
4 small courgettes [zucchini],
trimmed, washed and cut into
¼-inch slices

1 large red pepper, de-seeded and
sliced
1½ lb. sweet potato, peeled and
diced into 1-inch cubes
3 tomatoes, blanched, peeled,
seeded and chopped
2 medium-sized bananas, sliced
2 oz. canned pineapple chunks,
drained
1 teaspoon ground coriander
½ teaspoon ground cardamom
½ teaspoon ground fenugreek
½ teaspoon turmeric
¼ teaspoon hot chilli powder
3 tablespoons water
10 fl. oz. [1¼ cups] vegetable
stock
1-inch slice creamed coconut

Melt the butter or margarine in a
large saucepan over moderate heat.
When the foam subsides, add the
onions, garlic, chilli, courgettes
[zucchini], red pepper and sweet
potato. Cook them, stirring
occasionally, for 10 minutes.
Add the tomatoes, bananas and
pineapple chunks and cook, stirring
frequently, for 3 minutes.
Combine the coriander, cardamom,
fenugreek, turmeric and chilli powder
with the water in a small bowl to
make a smooth paste.
Stir the spice mixture into the fruit
and vegetable mixture, then pour in
the vegetable stock. Increase the
heat to high and bring the stock to
the boil. Reduce the heat to low,
cover the pan and simmer for 15
minutes, or until the vegetables are
cooked.
Stir in the creamed coconut, mixing
until it dissolves and the liquid
thickens. Simmer for a further 2
minutes.
Remove the pan from the heat and
turn the curry into a warmed serving
dish. Serve immediately.

Jerusalem artichokes flavoured with rosemary

Jerusalem artichokes should never be
overcooked, and this recipe
tastes best if the vegetables
retain a crunchy texture.
Preparation and cooking time:
30 minutes
SERVES 4

1½ lb. Jerusalem artichokes
1 tablespoon flour
2 tablespoons vinegar
water

sea salt
3 tablespoons butter
2 sprigs fresh rosemary, chopped *or* 1 sprig dried rosemary

Scrub the artichokes carefully and peel them very thinly. Reserve until cooking time in water to which 1 tablespoon flour and 2 tablespoonfuls vinegar have been added.
(This prevents discolouration.)
When ready to cook, cut the artichokes in thick slices and place in a saucepan with just enough water to cover and a little salt. Boil until soft but not mushy and then strain.
Melt the butter in a saucepan, add the artichokes and rosemary, and shake the pan to prevent sticking.
Warm the artichokes through, and serve completely covered with the butter and rosemary mixture.

Moroccan vegetable couscous

Serve this exotic dish with a light salad, crusty brown bread and lots of cool beer or white wine.
If you do not have a couscoussier, you can construct a temporary one by placing a colander lined with cheesecloth on top of a saucepan and sealing the space between the colander and the rim of the pan with a twisted, damp cloth.
Preparation and cooking time:
$3\frac{1}{4}$ hours
SERVES 6

1 lb. couscous
18 fl. oz. [$2\frac{1}{4}$ cups] lukewarm salted water
6 medium-sized courgettes [zucchini], trimmed, washed and sliced in half crosswise, then sliced in half lengthways
2 large green peppers, cored, de-seeded and sliced
2 large onions, quartered
3 medium-sized potatoes, scrubbed and sliced
1 small turnip, peeled and sliced
4 large carrots, scraped and quartered
3 pints [$7\frac{1}{2}$ cups] cold water
3 oz. [$\frac{3}{8}$ cup] butter *or* margarine, melted
1 lb. canned chick-peas, drained
4 oz. [$\frac{2}{3}$ cup] seedless raisins
2 oz. [$\frac{1}{3}$ cup] blanched almonds
1 lb. tomatoes, quartered
3 garlic cloves, crushed
3 green chillis, seeds removed and finely chopped
2 teaspoons sea salt
1 teaspoon freshly ground black pepper
$\frac{1}{2}$ teaspoon cayenne pepper
2 teaspoons ground cumin
2 teaspoons paprika
$\frac{1}{2}$ teaspoon ground saffron, dissolved in 1 teaspoon hot water
3 teaspoons turmeric
2 teaspoons ground coriander

Put the couscous grains into a large mixing bowl. Pour over 16 fluid ounces [2 cups] of the lukewarm water. Leave the couscous to soak for 1 hour, or until it swells slightly. Drain the grains in a fine strainer and set them aside.
Meanwhile, put the courgettes [zucchini], green peppers, onions, potatoes, turnip and carrots into the bottom half of the couscoussier. Pour in 2 pints [5 cups] of the cold water and bring the water to the boil over moderately high heat. Reduce the heat to low, cover the pan and simmer the vegetables for 30 minutes.
Fit the top half, or steamer, on to the couscoussier and pour the couscous grains into the steamer. Cover the pan and cook the mixture for 40 minutes.
Remove the top half, or steamer, from the couscoussier and transfer the couscous grains to a large mixing bowl. Pour on the melted butter or margarine and remaining lukewarm salted water. Leave the mixture to soak for 15 minutes.
Meanwhile, add the chick-peas, raisins, almonds and tomatoes to the bottom half of the couscoussier and pour in the remaining 1 pint [$2\frac{1}{2}$ cups] of cold water. Stir in the garlic, chillis, salt, pepper and spices. Bring the liquid to the boil over moderately high heat. Reduce the heat to low and simmer the mixture for 15 minutes.
Stir the couscous grains, breaking up any lumps that have formed and return the couscous to the top part, or steamer, of the couscoussier. Fit this attachment to the couscoussier again, cover and cook the mixture for a further 20 minutes.
Remove the couscoussier from the heat and take off the top half. Arrange the vegetable mixture in a large, deep serving dish and spoon on some of the cooking liquid. Reserve about 4 fluid ounces [$\frac{1}{2}$ cup] of the cooking liquid and discard the rest.
Put the couscous grains into a second serving dish and pour over the reserved cooking liquid. Serve at once.

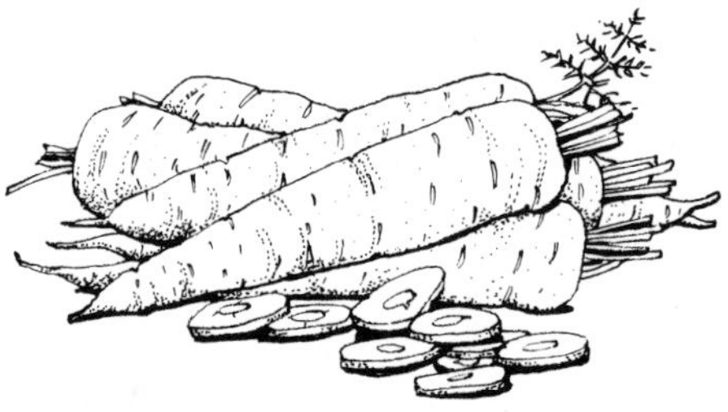

Sweet and sour carrots

This is a very different way to prepare a homely but delicious vegetable. Serve it as an accompaniment to risottos or omelettes.
Preparation and cooking time:
40 minutes
SERVES 4

1 lb. carrots, scraped and sliced
$1\frac{1}{2}$ pints [$3\frac{3}{4}$ cups] water
$\frac{1}{2}$ teaspoon salt
$1\frac{1}{2}$ oz. [3 tablespoons] butter or margarine
2 tablespoons flour
1 tablespoon honey
1 tablespoon wine vinegar
1 tablespoon chopped fresh parsley

Put the carrots into a large saucepan. Pour in the water and add the salt. Place the pan over moderately high heat and bring the water to the boil. Reduce the heat to moderate and cook the carrots for 10 to 15 minutes, or until they are tender. Drain the carrots and reserve 12 fluid ounces [$1\frac{1}{2}$ cups] of the cooking liquid.
Melt the butter or margarine over moderate heat in a medium-sized saucepan. Remove the pan from the heat and, with a wooden spoon, stir in the flour to make a smooth paste. Gradually add the reserved cooking liquid, stirring constantly.
Return the pan to the heat and cook the sauce stirring constantly, for 3 to 4 minutes, or until it is smooth and fairly thick. Stir in the honey and vinegar.
Add the carrots to the pan and continue to cook for 2 minutes, basting the carrots well with the sauce.
Turn the carrots and sauce into a warmed serving dish. Sprinkle the parsley over the carrots and serve.

Curry Creole (recipe page 97) is a delicious blend of fruit and vegetables that makes a meal on its own.

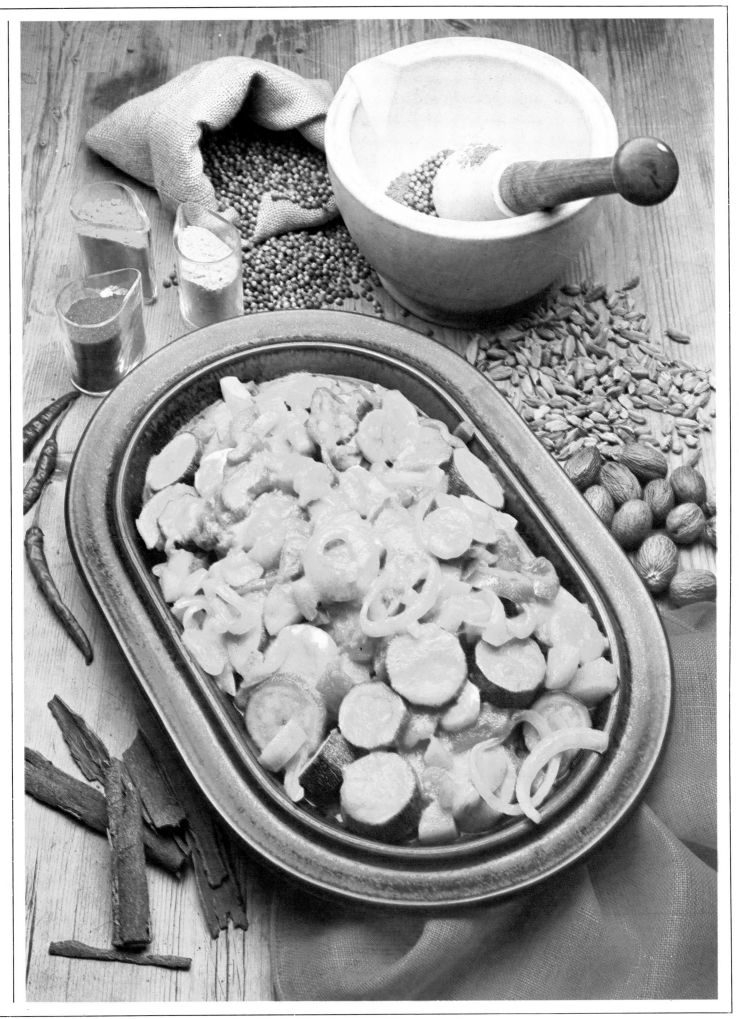

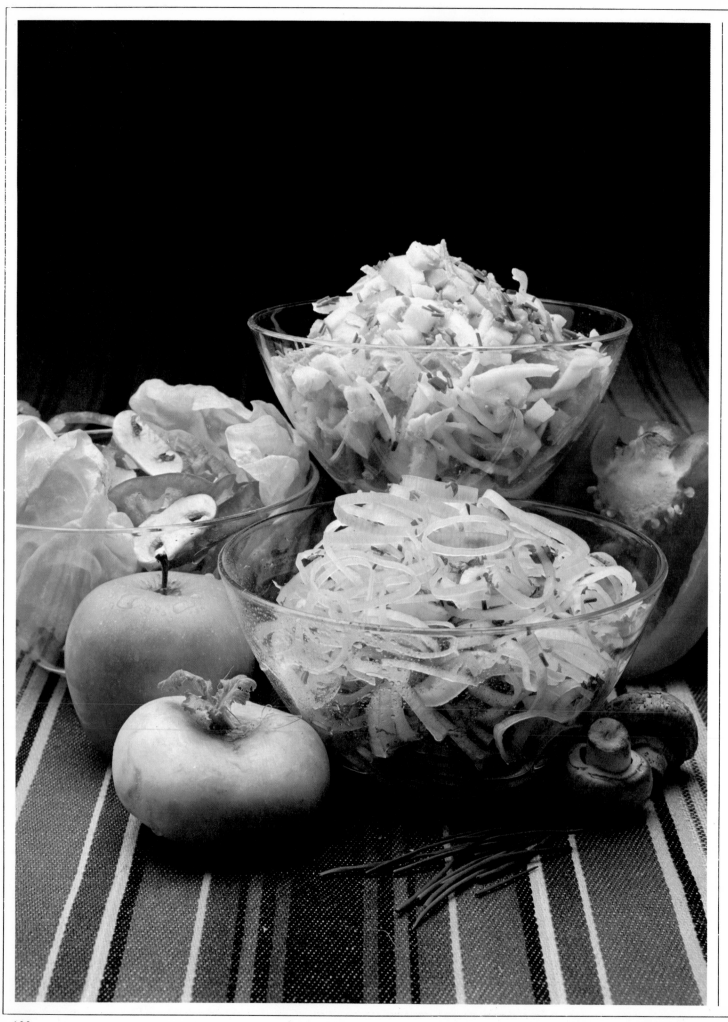

raw foods

Food is usually cooked to make it easier to chew and digest, and more appetizing to look at. But some foods taste and look just as good uncooked, particularly fruits and vegetables. And by serving green vegetables raw, much of the valuable vitamin C is preserved —instead of being washed away with the vegetable water. Many vegetables are delicious chopped and served in salad form: carrots, cucumber, cauliflower, mushrooms and cabbage all lend themselves well to this.

Combine raw fruits and vegetables to make interesting salads. Herbs, lemon juice and sometimes natural yogurt can also be added to improve the flavour. And nuts and raisins will add not only extra food value but also variety of taste and texture.

Health drinks

Fruit juices and vegetable drinks can supply valuable vitamins and variety, to your diet. A blender is, therefore, a good investment if you're slimming. But if you do not have a blender, you can squeeze fruits, or simmer vegetables in a little water, then press them through a sieve and allow to cool. Experiment with unusual herbs and vegetables for juices; they can be very good for you. Parsley juice, for example, is a rich source of vitamins A and C, and one of the few plants in which both these vitamins are present. Watercress juice supplies these vitamins too, plus iron and calcium. Cabbage juice or cabbage water is a particularly good base for a vegetable juice cocktail, and supplies vitamins A and C, calcium and iron. But the most nutritious of all is carrot juice. The juice of just four ounces of carrots supplies about half a day's requirements of Vitamin A, plus calcium, iodine, potassium, sulphur and sodium.

All fruit and vegetable juices taste better chilled. But drink them immediately they are brought into room temperature otherwise microscopic fungi will begin the work of fermentation, and impair the flavour.

Leek, cole slaw and peppery salads all look as good as they taste.

Beansprout salad
Mix drained, canned beansprouts with sliced mushrooms, firm tomato wedges, and chopped celery. Toss in lemon juice.

Brussels sprout salad
Mix shredded young sprouts with grated carrots, chopped celery, cauliflower sprigs, and chopped chives.

Celery salad
Mix shredded celery with shredded raw red or white cabbage, chopped onions, diced unpeeled eating apple and mustard and cress. Toss in a little yogurt mixed with horseradish for added piquancy.

Cole slaw salad
Mix shredded white cabbage with an equal quantity of shredded carrot, a diced apple and some natural, unsweetened yogurt. Add a few chives and a squeeze of lemon juice.

Crispy salad
Combine finely-shredded white cabbage, a few sprigs of cauliflower, chopped celery, sliced button mushrooms and a few almonds with a dressing of unsweetened tomato juice, tarragon vinegar and soy sauce. Leave to stand in a cool place, then cover with a few sliced mushrooms and capers and serve.

Leek salad
Slice some well-washed leeks finely and break them into rings. Mix with chopped chives and parsley and toss in lemon juice.

Mushroom and onion salad
Slice mushrooms and combine with grated onion and a little mild mustard. Add a few chopped tomatoes and garnish with cayenne pepper.

Peppery salad
Make a dressing with tomato juice, Worcestershire sauce and wine vinegar. Slice red, yellow or green peppers and a few mushrooms. Toss in the dressing and garnish with lettuce leaves.

Turnip salad
Peel and slice a small turnip and mix with shredded white cabbage, carrots, watercress, and sliced tomatoes.

Watercress and carrot salad
Mix chopped young carrots with watercress, chives, diced cucumber and a little chopped onion.

Beetroot [Beet] and parsley salad

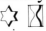

Beetroot [beets] can be very dull when served only in sharp malt vinegar. A sweeter dressing brings out their flavour, especially when combined with parsley and grated orange zest.
Preparation time: *10 minutes*
S E R V E S 4

1 lb. cooked beetroot [beets]
2 teaspoons grated orange zest
2 tablespoons chopped parsley
For the dressing:
4 fl. oz. [½ cup] olive or corn oil
2 tablespoons wine vinegar or lemon juice
1 teaspoon honey
sea salt
freshly ground black pepper

Peel and dice the beetroot [beets]. *Combine* the ingredients for the dressing and mix well. Toss the beetroot [beets] in the dressing and scatter parsley and grated orange zest over it before serving.

Crunchy winter salad

There is no need to cut down on health-giving salads in the winter. This one has a delicious blend of flavours and an agreeable crunchy texture. The proportions of the ingredients may be altered according to availability.
Preparation time: *15 minutes*
S E R V E S 4

½ medium-sized firm white cabbage
1 small bulb fennel
2 medium carrots
1 eating apple
½ medium-sized green pepper
2 tablespoons cashew nuts
2 tablespoons raisins
6-8 sprigs parsley
1 medium onion (optional)
For the dressing:
4 fl. oz. [½ cup] olive or corn oil
2 tablespoons wine vinegar
1 teaspoon clear honey
sea salt
freshly ground black pepper

Remove outer leaves from the cabbage. Trim the fennel. Scrape the carrots, peel, quarter and core the apple. Wash, core and de-seed the pepper. *Shred* the cabbage finely with a sharp knife, chop the fennel, apple and pepper. Grate carrots and nuts.

Mix all dressing ingredients, beat together and season to taste. Toss the shredded vegetables in the dressing, mix with nuts and raisins and place in salad bowl.

Wash and dry the parsley, chop and scatter over the salad before serving. Top with the onion, cut into rings.

Mushroom and cucumber salad

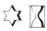

This unusual and flavoursome salad can be made at any time of the year.
Preparation time: *15 minutes*
SERVES 4

1 small cucumber
4 oz. mushrooms
1 medium-sized onion
3 slices stale wholemeal
  [wholewheat] **bread**
vegetable oil for frying
For the dressing:
4 fl. oz. [½ cup] **olive or corn oil**
2 tablespoons **wine vinegar**
sea salt
freshly ground black pepper
To garnish:
lettuce leaves

Peel and dice the cucumber. Wash, dry and slice the mushrooms. Peel the onion and cut into fine rings.
Beat together all the ingredients for the dressing.
Trim the crusts from the bread, cut into ½-inch cubes and fry in a little hot oil until crisp. Drain well.
Just before serving, toss the vegetables and croûtons well in the dressing and arrange on a bed of lettuce leaves.

Turkish salad

This tastes delicious with beef stew.
Preparation time: *45 minutes*
SERVES 4-6

1 cucumber
2-3 garlic cloves
15 fl. oz. [2 cups] **natural yogurt**
sea salt
freshly ground black pepper
2 tablespoons **chopped fresh mint**

Slice or dice the cucumber, sprinkle it with salt and leave for 30 minutes.
Crush the garlic into a bowl, mix in the yogurt and season to taste. Add the mint. Strain off the cucumber and add it to the yogurt mixture.

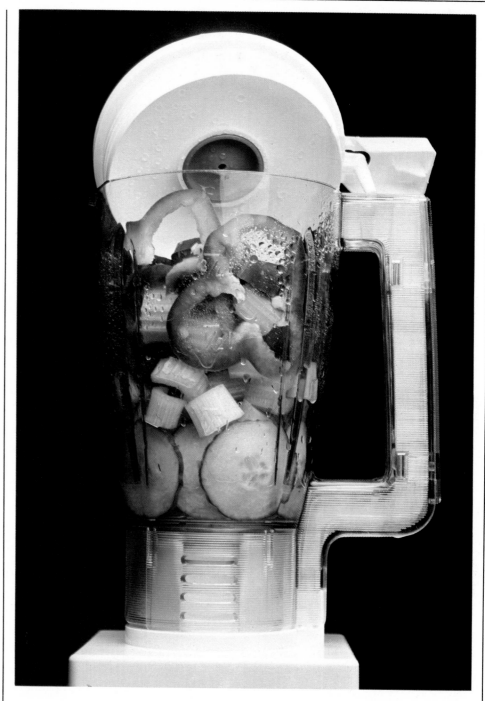

Celery, cucumber and green pepper combine for a health-giving drink.

Fruit juices

1. Equal parts strawberry and pineapple juice.
2. 1 cup apple juice, 1 cup blackberry juice and a teaspoon of honey.
3. 1 cup orange juice, 1 tablespoon cucumber juice, 1 tablespoon lemon juice.
4. 1 cup melon juice, 1 tablespoon orange juice and a dash of lemon juice. Mint and orange slices for garnish.
5. 1 cup apple juice, 1 tablespoon blackcurrant juice and 1 tablespoon natural, unsweetened yogurt.
6. 1 cup orange juice, 1 tablespoon peach juice, 1 teaspoon lime juice.

Vegetable juices

1. 1 cup tomato juice, 1 tablespoon lemon juice, and a dash of Worcestershire sauce.
2. Equal parts cabbage, carrot and parsley juice. Cucumber slices and paprika pepper as garnish.
3. 1 cup celery juice, 1 tablespoon parsley juice, 1 tablespoon carrot juice, chopped chives for garnish.
4. 5 fl. oz. [⅝ cup] natural, unsweetened yogurt, 4 fl. oz. [½ cup] tomato juice, and a squeeze of lemon juice.
5. Equal parts juice of celery, cucumber, and green pepper plus a teaspoonful of lemon juice.
6. 1 cup carrot juice, 1 tablespoon cabbage juice and 1 tablespoon turnip juice.

nuts for everybody

Nuts are not just for vegetarians. They provide an interesting addition to any diet and are also a valuable source of protein. To vary your menus, include a nut-based dish occasionally as an alternative to meat, fish, eggs or cheese. Remember, too, that a small packet of peanuts makes a nutritious protein-packed lunch-time snack when it is impossible to have a proper meal. Add nuts to fruit or salad vegetables and you get the bonus of vitamins B and C as well as protein. And if you have a glass of fresh milk as well you get a well-balanced meal without the trouble of cooking.

Brazil nuts provide almost as much protein gram for gram as roast chicken, and more than pork sausages or luncheon meat. So a Nut Bake (recipe over) could be better value for a summer lunch than sliced luncheon meat and salad. Health-food shops have a good choice of nuts—ground, mixed or whole. Try these recipes, then experiment with different tastes and different mixtures. Nut cookery is fun, and the results are delicious!

Do not leave nut cookery to vegetarians. Nut Rolls (recipe on next page) taste delicious and would make a change from a main meat dish.

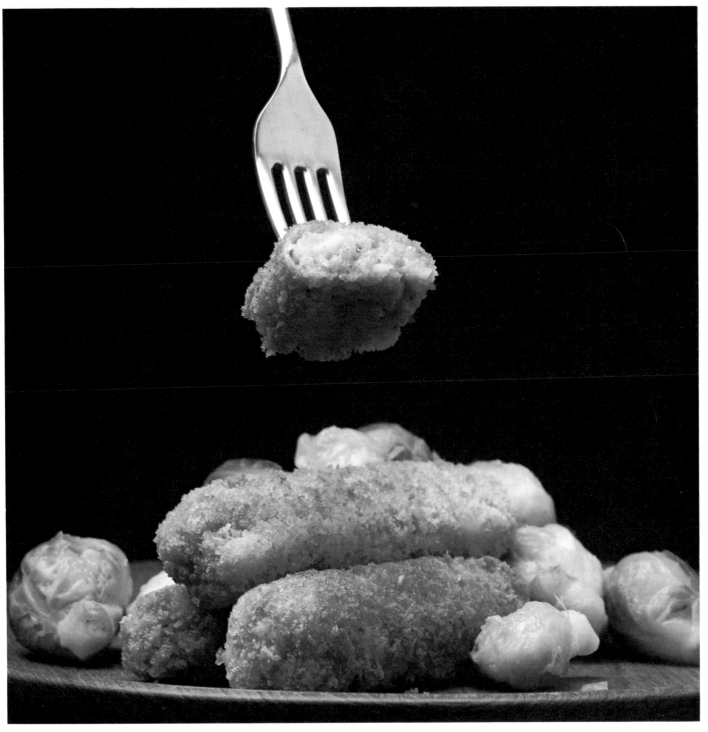

Foule Sudani

This nourishing peanut soup from
the Sudan is rich in protein and
vitamins.
Preparation and cooking time:
30 minutes
S E R V E S 4

1 oz. **salted peanuts**
3 oz. **unsalted peanuts**
2 tablespoons **ground nut oil**
2 medium-sized **onions, peeled and
  chopped**
½ **chicken stock cube, dissolved in
  1½ pints [3¾ cups] hot water
  or 1½ pints [3¾ cups] home-made
  stock**
freshly ground black pepper
salt

Grind the peanuts in a coffee mill or
blender, (a little at a time,
otherwise the mill clogs up).
Heat the oil in a large heavy-bottomed
pan over moderate heat. Fry the onions
in the oil until golden brown.
Add the stock to the pan with the
ground peanuts, bring to the boil,
then reduce the heat and simmer for
10 minutes.
Remove the pan from the heat. Transfer
the contents of the pan to a blender
or food mill and blend thoroughly,
then re-heat.
Season with pepper and salt to taste.
(If you use a stock cube, this soup
does not normally need extra salt.)

Hazelnut pear salad

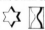

This aromatic salad with its
unusual combination of flavours
makes a filling luncheon dish.
Preparation time:
15 minutes
S E R V E S 4

4 large **pears**
2 teaspoons **lemon juice**
8 oz. **cottage cheese**
4 oz. [⅔ cup] **hazelnuts, coarsely
  chopped**
2 teaspoons **finely chopped sweet
  cicely (optional)**
1 teaspoon **finely chopped lemon
  balm (optional)**
6 **lettuce leaves**

Peel the pears, halve them and
remove the cores. Chop the flesh
into a medium-sized mixing bowl.
Sprinkle the lemon juice over the pears.

Stir in the cottage cheese and
hazelnuts, with the sweet cicely and
lemon balm if you are using them.
Arrange the lettuce leaves on a
shallow serving dish. Pile the pear
mixture in the centre and serve.

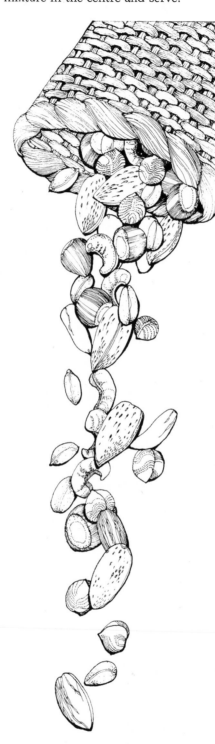

Nut bake

This unusual savoury is suitable for
a main course or supper dish. Serve
it accompanied by green vegetables
or a salad and wholemeal [wholewheat]
bread. Any nuts except peanuts can
be used.

Preparation and cooking time:
1 hour
S E R V E S 4

8 oz. [1⅓ cups] **grated nuts**
8 oz. **tomatoes, skinned and sliced**
1 small **onion, finely chopped**
2 **eggs, beaten**
sea salt
1 teaspoon **mixed chopped thyme
  and marjoram, fresh or dried**

Heat the oven to 400°F (Gas Mark 6,
205°C).
Mix together the nuts, tomatoes and
onions. Add the eggs, stir well, then
add the salt and herbs.
Grease an ovenproof dish, put in the
nut mixture, and bake in the oven
for 30-40 minutes until well-risen
and golden on the top.

Nut rolls

This tasty dish can be eaten hot or
cold and is very good for a picnic
or snack lunch. Any type of nuts
except peanuts can be used.
Preparation and cooking time:
40 minutes
S E R V E S 4

2 oz. [4 tablespoons] **butter or lard**
2 oz. wholemeal [½ cup wholewheat]
  flour
1 pint [2½ cups] **stock or water**
sea salt
¼ teaspoon **chopped marjoram**
¼ teaspoon **chopped thyme**
1 teaspoon **yeast extract**
4 oz. wholemeal [2 cups wholewheat]
  breadcrumbs
2 oz. [⅓ cup] **nuts, grated**
1 **egg**
2 tablespoons **milk**

Melt the fat in a saucepan over
moderate heat. Add the flour and
cook gently for 2 minutes, stirring
continuously. Add the stock, salt,
herbs and yeast extract, mix well
and cook for 5 minutes stirring all
the time.
Take the pan off the heat, add 3
ounces [1½ cups] of the breadcrumbs
and all the nuts. Mix well, leave to
cool and then form into sausage-
shaped rolls.
Beat together the egg and the milk.
Dip the nut rolls into this mixture,
and then cover them with the
remaining breadcrumbs.
Fry in deep fat for about 10 minutes
or until golden brown. Drain on
absorbent kitchen paper.

rice

It is difficult to obtain an ample supply of vitamin B2 (riboflavin) in the average Western diet. The usual recommended daily requirement for tip-top health is one to three milligrams, but many nutritionists feel that about four to five milligrams would be a good level. An average portion of liver, or eight small glasses of milk, would supply this required amount but few people eat liver regularly or drink much milk in one day.

It is, therefore, wise to substitute vitamin B rich foods for other foods whenever practical. And about 1 cup of brown rice can add .02 milligrams of vitamin B2, plus the other valuable members of the B family. It is also a versatile accompaniment to many other foods and delicious in its own right. (White, polished rice has the brown husk and germ removed. It supplies very little vitamin B and less vitamin E.) Some recipes are given below, but remember that the rice can be enjoyed just on its own. The nutty taste is far more interesting than that of plain boiled white rice. Use it instead of potatoes, with cold salads or mixed with chopped vegetables and herbs.

Brown rice does, however, take longer to cook. One method is as follows: rinse the rice under the tap in a wire strainer, bring three cups water to boiling point in a large saucepan, add the cup of rice and boil for 5 minutes. Turn down the heat and simmer for 20 minutes. Turn off the heat, add seasoning and leave the rice to stand for about one hour until the remaining water is absorbed. Warm through just before serving.

Avocado rice salad

Unpolished rice is delicious in salads. This one may be used on its own as a first course, or as an accompaniment to cold meats.
Preparation time:
40 minutes
S E R V E S 4

1 small lettuce
2 oz. [⅓ cup] **long-grain unpolished rice**

1 ripe avocado pear
1 lemon
1 small onion
3-inch piece of cucumber
½ **green pepper**
2 ripe tomatoes, sliced
For the dressing:
4 fl. oz. [½ cup] **olive or corn oil**
2 tablespoons wine vinegar
½ **teaspoon clear honey**
sea salt
freshly ground black pepper

Wash the lettuce, pat dry and crisp in the refrigerator.
Cook the rice in boiling, salted water until just tender but not mushy. Strain in a sieve and rinse well under cold running water. Drain and dry.
Halve the avocado pear, scoop out the flesh and dice. Cut the lemon in half and squeeze the juice from one half. Toss the avocado flesh in the lemon juice. Peel and dice the onion and cucumber. De-seed and chop the pepper.
Combine the ingredients for the dressing and beat well. Toss the vegetables and rice in the dressing, arrange on lettuce leaves in a salad bowl or on small dishes. Top with sliced tomato and the remaining half lemon, sliced.

Brazilian rice

This Brazilian method of cooking rice is both simple and tasty.
Preparation and cooking time:
45 minutes
S E R V E S 4

4 tablespoons olive oil
1 large onion, thinly sliced
12 oz. [2 cups] **long-grain brown rice, washed, soaked in cold water for 30 minutes and drained**
2 tomatoes, blanched, peeled and chopped
1 teaspoon sea salt
1¼ pints [3 cups] boiling water

Heat the oil over moderate heat in a large saucepan. Add the onion and fry it, stirring occasionally, for 5 to 7

minutes, or until it is soft and translucent but not brown. Add the rice and fry for 5 minutes, stirring constantly.
Stir in the tomatoes and salt. Cook for 2 minutes and then pour in the boiling water.
Reduce the heat to low, cover the pan and simmer for 15 to 20 minutes, or until the rice is tender and all the liquid has been absorbed.
Turn the rice into a warmed serving dish and serve immediately.

Chicken liver pilaff

This nutritious main course can be cooked in advance and reheated. Serve it with a green salad.
Preparation and cooking time:
50 minutes
S E R V E S 4

6 oz. [1 cup] **brown rice**
1 pint [2½ cups] **water**
1½ teaspoons salt
3 tablespoons vegetable oil
1 medium-sized onion, chopped
3 celery stalks, chopped
4 oz. mushrooms, sliced
8 oz. chicken liver, cut in half
½ teaspoon basil
a pinch of nutmeg
½ teaspoon wholemeal [wholewheat] flour
1 tablespoon yeast extract
To garnish:
parsley, chopped

Put the rice, water, 1 teaspoon of salt and 1 tablespoon of the oil into a large saucepan. Bring to the boil then reduce heat and simmer for 45 minutes or until the rice is tender and all the liquid absorbed.
Heat the remaining oil in a large frying pan and sauté the onions, celery, mushrooms and livers in it for 5-7 minutes or until the vegetables and liver are tender. Add the rest of the seasonings, flour and yeast extract. Cook for 1 minute stirring continuously. Add the cooked rice and heat through thoroughly.
Garnish with chopped parsley and serve.

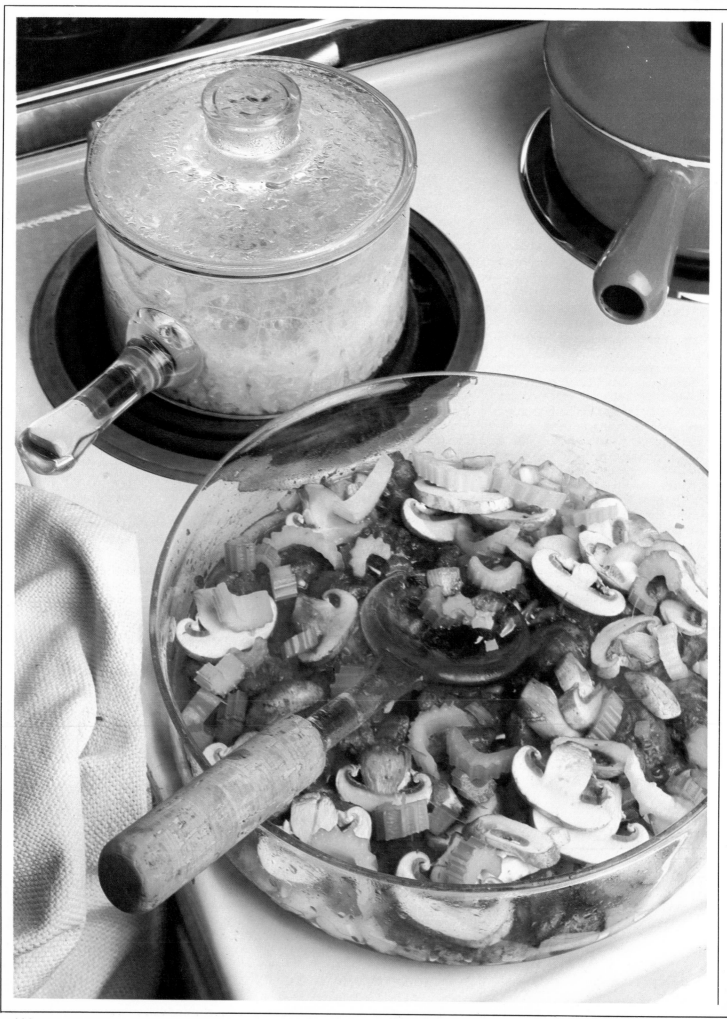

Rice and salmon or tuna salad

This salad is delicious served with a yogurt dressing (see page 96) and wholemeal [wholewheat] bread. The ingredients and proportions can be slightly modified.
Preparation and cooking time:
1½ hours
S E R V E S 4

1 tablespoon vegetable oil
6 oz. [1 cup] brown rice
1 small onion finely chopped
1 pint [2½ cups] water
1 teaspoon sea salt
8 oz. canned salmon or tuna fish
1 crisp eating apple (tossed in lemon juice to prevent discoloration)
2 medium-sized carrots, grated coarsely
2 oz. [½ cup] cabbage, shredded
2 oz. [½ cup] walnuts, coarsely chopped
To garnish:
1 bunch watercress
4 medium-sized tomatoes, sliced

Heat the oil in a pan and sauté the rice and onion in it for 2 minutes. Add the water and the salt, bring to the boil and simmer, with the lid on the pan, for about 45 minutes or until the rice and onion are tender and the water is absorbed. Set on one side and leave to cool.
Drain the oil from the fish, and flake the flesh.
Mix the rice together with the prepared vegetables. Add the flaked fish and mix well using a kitchen fork to help separate the ingredients.
Heap on to a salad dish, garnish with watercress and tomato slices, and serve.

Rice with chicken and cherries

An exotic and unusual combination of tastes, Chicken and Cherries is an adaptation of an Iranian dish.
Preparation and cooking time:
1½ hours
S E R V E S 4

1 x 3 lb. chicken, cut into 8 serving pieces

Chicken Liver Pilaff is easy to prepare and makes a good dinner party dish.

2 teaspoons sea salt
1 teaspoon finely ground black pepper
4 tablespoons olive oil
2 medium-sized onions, finely sliced
3 fl. oz. [⅜ cup] chicken stock
1½ lb. fresh black Morello cherries, stoned or 2 lb. canned Morello cherries, drained and stoned
2 oz. [¼ cup] sugar
2 tablespoons water
12 oz. [2 cups] long-grain rice, washed and drained
4 oz. [½ cup] butter, melted
½ teaspoon crushed saffron threads, dissolved in 1 tablespoon hot water

On a chopping board, sprinkle the chicken pieces with the salt and pepper and set aside.
In a large frying-pan heat the oil over moderate heat. When it is hot, add the chicken pieces, a few at a time. Cook them for 5 to 7 minutes on each side or until they are evenly and thoroughly browned.
When the chicken is browned, transfer it to a heated plate. Add the onions to the oil remaining in the frying-pan and fry them for 6 minutes, or until they begin to brown slightly.
Return the chicken pieces to the frying-pan, pour in the chicken stock and bring the mixture to the boil. Reduce the heat to low, cover the pan and cook the chicken for 30 minutes, or until it is tender when pierced with a fork.
While the chicken is simmering, combine the cherries, sugar and water together in a medium-sized saucepan over low heat. Stirring frequently, simmer uncovered for 5 minutes or until the sugar has dissolved and most of the cherry liquid has evaporated. Remove from heat and set aside.
In a large saucepan, bring 2½ pints [3¾ cups] of water to the boil over moderate heat. Add the rice and boil for 5 minutes. Remove the pan from the heat and drain the rice through a strainer. Set aside.
Transfer the chicken pieces to a plate, reserving about 2 tablespoons of the cooking liquid and the browned onion slices.
Put the reserved cooking liquid and half melted butter into a large flame-proof casserole and mix well. Place half of the rice on the bottom of the casserole, spreading it out evenly, and cook over moderate heat for 8 minutes. Remove the casserole from the heat. Add the chicken pieces, onions and about half of the cherries.

Arrange the remainder of the rice on top of the mixture. Pour in the remaining cherries with their cooking liquid, cover the casserole and simmer over very low heat for 15 minutes or until the rice is tender.
Remove about 4 ounces [1 cup] of the cooked rice from the casserole and place it in a medium-sized bowl. Add the remainder of the melted butter and the dissolved saffron threads to the rice. Stir well. Set aside.
Arrange half the remaining rice in the casserole on the base of a serving platter and place the chicken pieces with the onions on top. Cover the meat with the cherries and the remaining rice and sprinkle the saffron rice on top and around the edge.

Vegetable pilaff

Served with fried chicken this makes an excellent family lunch or supper dish.
Preparation and cooking time:
45 minutes
S E R V E S 4-6

2 fl. oz. [¼ cup] vegetable oil
4 medium-sized carrots, scraped and sliced
4 medium-sized onions, 3 thinly sliced and 1 sliced and pushed out into rings
2 medium-sized potatoes, sliced
9 oz. [1½ cups] long-grain brown rice, washed, soaked in cold water for 30 minutes and drained
1 teaspoon sea salt
1 teaspoon freshly ground black pepper
1 teaspoon dried dill leaves
1 pint [2½ cups] water
8 fl. oz. [1 cup] vegetable stock

Heat the oil in a large saucepan over moderate heat. When the oil is hot, add the carrots, the three sliced onions and the potatoes. Cook, stirring occasionally, for 8 minutes, or until the vegetables have softened but are not brown. Stir in the rice and, stirring constantly, cook for 2 minutes.
Stir in the salt, pepper and dill. Add the stock and the water and increase the heat to high. Bring the mixture to the boil. Reduce the heat to low, cover the pan and simmer for 20 to 25 minutes, or until the rice is tender and all the liquid has been absorbed.
Transfer the mixture to a deep serving dish. Scatter the onion rings on top and serve immediately.

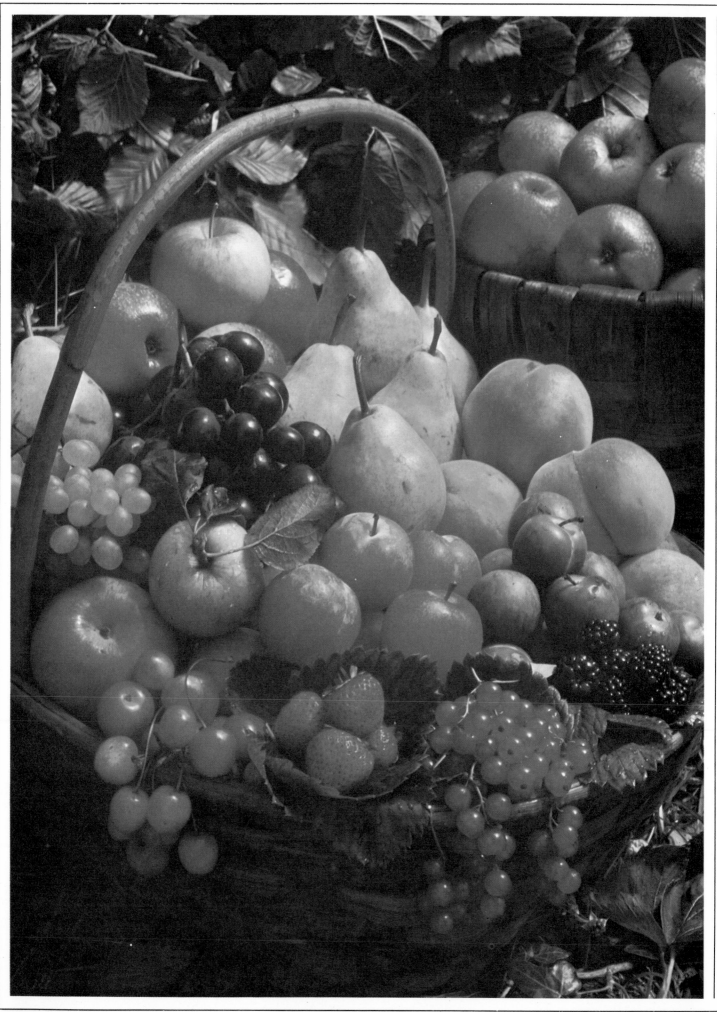

fresh & dried fruits

Roughage, vitamin C, vitamin B, and natural sugars are all supplied by fruits. To give balance and nourishment every meal should include a fresh fruit, fruit juice or fruit-based dessert. Children should be encouraged to enjoy fresh fruits and offered fruit as the ideal between-meals snack. And if you cannot persuade the men in the family to eat fruit raw, then serve it in the guise of tasty, filling pies and puddings.

Add fruits to salads and meat dishes. Orange segments go well with liver as well as with the traditional duck, apples are the classic accompaniment to pork, pineapple tastes marvellous with ham. Buy fruits with care. Look for firm, fresh apples and pears, unbruised bananas, plump succulent soft fruits. If you grow your own fruit pick it at the last minute before cooking or deep-freeze it quickly for future use.

Keep a good supply of dried fruits like apricots, figs and dates. These are useful for desserts and for simple, but delicious, fruit compôtes which taste marvellous with honey and fresh cream.

Coconut apples

⋈ ⋈

Baked apples are delicious with a sweet filling. This one is made with creamy coconut and iron-rich apricots.
Preparation and cooking time:
1 hour 20 minutes
S E R V E S 4

4 large cooking apples
2 oz. [⅓ cup] dried apricots
4 oz. creamed coconut, available from speciality shops
2 oz. [½ cup] stale cake crumbs
3 tablespoons honey
5 fl. oz. [⅝ cup] water

Heat the oven to 350°F (Gas Mark 4, 180°C).
Wash the apples well and core them, replacing the section of core from the base as a 'stopper' for the filling.

Pour boiling water over the apricots, leave for 10 minutes, then drain them and snip or chop into small pieces.
Meanwhile, put the creamed coconut through a coarse mill or grinder, combine half with the cake crumbs and 2 tablespoons of the honey. Stir in the chopped apricots and stuff the apples with the mixture. Make a slit with a sharp knife round the middle of each apple to prevent bursting.
Place the apples in a shallow baking dish. Pour the remaining tablespoon of honey and the water around them and cook for 1 hour or until apples are soft. Baste occasionally and add more water and honey if necessary.
Serve hot or cold, with the rest of the coconut beaten to a cream with a little water.

Date and orange salad

⋈ ⋈

This light, refreshing dessert is ideal to round off a substantial meal. It may be served alone or with cream, sour cream or yogurt.
Preparation and cooking time:
1 hour, plus chilling time
S E R V E S 4

4 oz. [⅔ cup] dried figs
½ tablespoon soft brown sugar
3 large oranges
12 dessert dates
4 tablespoons maple syrup

Wash the figs well. Put them in a pan with the sugar. Add enough boiling water to cover. Soak for 30 minutes, then simmer gently for 5 minutes. Remove the figs with a perforated spoon. Boil up liquid and reduce slightly. Cool and reserve.
Peel the oranges, remove all pith and slice thinly with a sharp knife. Arrange in a shallow serving dish.
Stone the dates. Snip stems from figs. Chop the fruit roughly and scatter over oranges. Spoon the maple syrup over, together with 2 tablespoons reserved syrup from the figs.
Chill lightly before serving.

Fig and apple pie

⋈ ⋈

Apple pie is a favourite standby, and it is a good idea to have a new version sometimes to offer hungry families.

Preparation and cooking time:
1 hour 10 minutes
S E R V E S 4

8 oz. dried figs
8 oz. cooking apples
2 tablespoons soft brown sugar
4 tablespoons marmalade
For the pastry:
8 oz. [2 cups] flour
pinch of sea salt
4 oz. [½ cup] margarine
water

Heat the oven to 425°F (Gas Mark 7, 220°C).
Meanwhile, wash the figs well, cover with boiling water and leave to soak for 30 minutes.
Sift the flour and salt together, rub in margarine and add just enough water to make a firm dough. Roll out and use half to line a greased pie plate.
Peel, core and slice the apples. Drain the figs and snip off their stalks. Chop roughly. Place the figs in the pie plate with the apples, sprinkle with sugar and top with the marmalade. Roll out the remaining pastry, cover pie, seal and trim the edges.
Bake for 15 minutes, then lower heat to 350°F (Gas Mark 4, 180°C) for a further 15-20 minutes, or until the pie crust is golden brown.

Strawberries with caramel topping

⋈ ⋈

This is a light summer dessert to make when strawberries are at their best.
Preparation and cooking time:
15 minutes, plus 1 hour chilling time
S E R V E S 4

1 lb. ripe strawberries
2 tablespoons soft brown sugar
grated zest of 1 orange
10 fl. oz. [1¼ cups] natural yogurt
2-4 oz. demerara [¼-½ cup light brown] sugar

Hull and wash the strawberries. Drain and pat dry. Toss in the soft brown sugar and arrange in a shallow fireproof dish.
Heat the grill [broiler].
Mix the orange zest into the yogurt and spread over the strawberries. Sprinkle the demerara sugar over the yogurt in an even layer and place under the hot grill [broiler] until the sugar melts. Cool the dish.
Chill for 1 hour, so that the sugar forms a crisp caramel topping.

beans & lentils

Beans are not only cheap and filling they are also a rich source of protein, vitamins and minerals (sodium, potassium, magnesium, phosphorus, sulphur). By adding lentils, soya or kidney beans to a meat dish or soup you effectively double the nutritional value of the dish. So when budgeting is difficult it is a good idea to choose cheaper cuts of meat and add beans to give more nourishment to the finished dish. Always keep dried beans in your store-cupboard for a good standby when a hot, tasty main course or soup is required.

Remember that all dried pulses need soaking overnight before use. Use a good-sized pot and make sure the water level is double the depth of the beans.

Braised beef rolls with beans

This is a delicious way of cooking the less expensive cuts of beef. These are just as nutritious as the more expensive cuts and this dish is made even more so by the addition of beans.
Preparation and cooking time:
3½ hours
S E R V E S 4

2 oz. [¼ cup] **red kidney beans, soaked overnight**
1½ lb. **lean braising steak**
4 slices **streaky bacon**
mustard to taste
4 oz. [⅔ cup] **prunes, soaked overnight**
2 tablespoons **vegetable oil**
2 **celery stalks**
2 oz. **mushrooms**
1 **medium-sized onion**
2 tablespoons **sea salt**
¼ teaspoon **freshly ground black pepper**
water or stock

Simmer the beans in fresh, unsalted water until tender (about 1½ hours). Drain and reserve.
Heat the oven to 350°F (Gas Mark 4, 180°C).
Trim the steak, beat it out until

very thin and divide into 8 slices. De-rind the bacon and cut each slice in half. Lay a piece on each beef slice and smear well with prepared mustard.
Drain the prunes, stone them and snip into small pieces with kitchen scissors. Divide among the beef slices. Form into rolls and secure with thin string or thread. Heat the oil in a pan and brown the rolls quickly.
Wash the celery and mushrooms, peel the onion. Chop vegetables roughly and place in a deep casserole. Set the beef rolls on the bed of chopped vegetables, add seasoning and pour about half an inch of water or stock into the bottom of the dish.
Cover and cook for 1-1½ hours or until the meat is tender, adding the beans to the dish for the last half hour of cooking. Snip the thread and remove carefully from the rolls before serving.

Lentil and onion pie

This is a good dish for cooks who like to use a pre-set oven. (Prepare the ingredients the night before the meal if you wish.) As it is very filling serve with a simple green vegetable or salad and follow it with fruit.
Preparation and cooking time:
1 hour, plus 12 hours soaking time for the lentils
S E R V E S 4

12 oz. **lentils**
8 oz. **potatoes**
milk
½ oz. [1 tablespoon] **butter**
1 large **onion**
1 lb. **tomatoes**
2 oz. [4 tablespoons] **lard or dripping**
1 **bay leaf**

Soak the lentils for 12 hours or overnight and cook them in a little water for 45 minutes or until soft. Strain and mash thoroughly, add the bay leaf and set aside.
Boil the potatoes in their skins, skin and mash thoroughly with a little milk and butter.
Chop the onion and tomatoes and stew until soft in half the lard.
Heat the oven to 375°F (Gas Mark 5, 190°C).
Grease an ovenproof dish. Put in the lentils, top with the tomato and onion mixture and add the mashed potatoes. Dot with the remaining fat and bake in the oven for 30 minutes.

Lentil stew

This delicious warming stew is useful as a supper dish for a hungry family and makes an excellent standby for times when meat is not available.
Preparation and cooking time:
1½ hours, plus 12 hours soaking time for lentils
S E R V E S 4

8 oz. **brown lentils**
1 **medium-sized carrot**
2 **leeks**
1 **celery stalk**
2 large **onions**
1 small **turnip**
3 oz. [⅜ cup] **lard or dripping**
1 oz. [¼ cup] **flour**
5 fl. oz. [⅝ cup] **stock**
sea salt
freshly-ground black pepper
To garnish:
parsley, chopped

Soak the lentils for 12 hours or overnight and cook them in a little water for about 45 minutes or until almost soft.
Meanwhile cut the vegetables into small pieces. Melt half the fat in a large pan and simmer the vegetables in it for 10 minutes.
Drain off any surplus water from the lentils and add them to the vegetables.
Cook for a further 5-10 minutes, stirring to prevent sticking.
Melt the rest of the fat in a large saucepan, add the flour, stir again then add the stock, stirring all the time to make a smooth sauce. Add the lentil and vegetable mixture, season to taste and serve garnished with chopped parsley.

Red bean salad

This makes an unusual addition to a cold buffet table or cold meat dish. You do, however, have to remember to soak the beans overnight in advance.
Preparation and cooking time:
2 hours
S E R V E S 2-4

4 oz. **dried red** *or* **brown beans, soaked overnight**
bouquet garni of 1 bay leaf, 1 celery stalk and 4-5 parsley sprigs
1 **medium-sized onion, finely sliced**

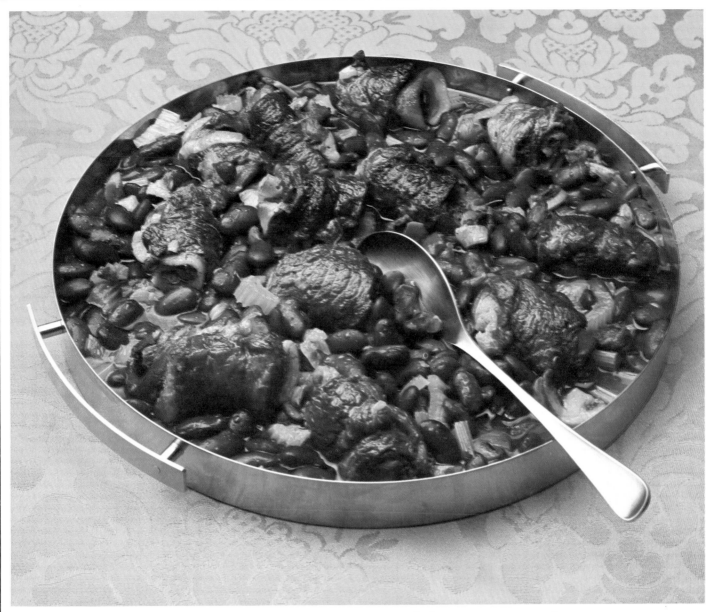

2 ripe firm tomatoes
2 oz. [½ cup] cheese, grated
2 tablespoons chopped parsley
sea salt
freshly ground black pepper
For the dressing:
2 fl. oz. [¼ cup] mayonnaise
2 fl. oz. double [¼ cup heavy]
  cream (lightly whipped)
the grated zest and juice of ¼ lemon
¼ teaspoon dry mustard
sea salt
freshly ground black pepper

Drain the beans. Put them in a large saucepan, cover with slightly salted water and bring to the boil very slowly. Add the bouquet garni. Cover the pan and simmer for 1 hour, or until the beans are tender, adding the onion 3-4 minutes before the end of the cooking time. Drain off the liquid and put the beans and onion into a bowl.
Scald, then skin the tomatoes. Cut them in half and remove the seeds and

Braised Beef Rolls with beans look colourful and are very nutritious.

core. Add them to the bean mixture, then add the cheese, parsley and seasoning to taste.
To make the dressing stir the cream into the mayonnaise. Slowly add the lemon zest and juice, stirring continuously. Add the mustard and season well. The dressing should be a thin consistency. If the mixture is thick add 1 tablespoon of warm water.
Mix the bean mixture with the dressing and serve.

Soya bean and green pepper salad

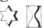

This nourishing, crunchy side salad is delicious with Cauliflower Cheese or a cheese omelette.
Preparation time:
20 minutes

SERVES 4

4 green peppers, de-seeded and cut
  into thin strips
6 spring onions [scallions],
  finely chopped
4 tablespoons olive oil
2 tablespoons dry red wine
½ garlic clove, finely chopped
½ teaspoon sea salt
¼ teaspoon freshly ground black
  pepper
4 tablespoons salted soya bean
  splits

Combine in a medium-sized salad bowl the green pepper strips and spring onions [scallions]. Set aside.
Combine the oil, wine, garlic, salt and pepper in a screw-top jar. Cover the jar and shake it for 10 seconds.
Pour this dressing over the green peppers and onions [scallions]. Toss the ingredients together thoroughly. Sprinkle over the soya bean splits and serve.

Dried beans and peas

These are the 'pulses'—dried vegetables which can be used instead of fresh ones when they are scarce, *or* as part of the main course, since they are rich in protein. Boiled lentils, for example, supply 6.8 grams of protein per 100 grams—which compares well with yogurt (4.7) and eggs (11.9).

The nutritional value of the pulse vegetables has long been recognized in hot countries round the Mediterranean, and in the Near, Middle and Far East. The fact that they can be stored for long periods without losing this value is a good point where the climate causes fresh foods to deteriorate quickly.

In France, the slow-cooking 'cassoulet'—a dish based on dried haricot beans—is a culinary classic. In Egypt, where lentils are eaten almost every day in most homes, rich spices are added to give piquancy to the fairly bland taste of the pulse vegetables.

In Russia and North East Europe, the larger brown lentils and brown beans are used for substantial family supper dishes. In Czechoslovakia, a winter soup is made from dried brown lentils soaked overnight, then cooked and sieved to make a purée. This is combined with grated onion, garlic, red pepper and rounds of smoked sausage. The result is appetizing and *very* filling—what's more, it is cheap too.

In the photograph, right, the beautiful yellows, browns and greens of the pulses make a rich mosaic of colour. Use the key below for easy identification:

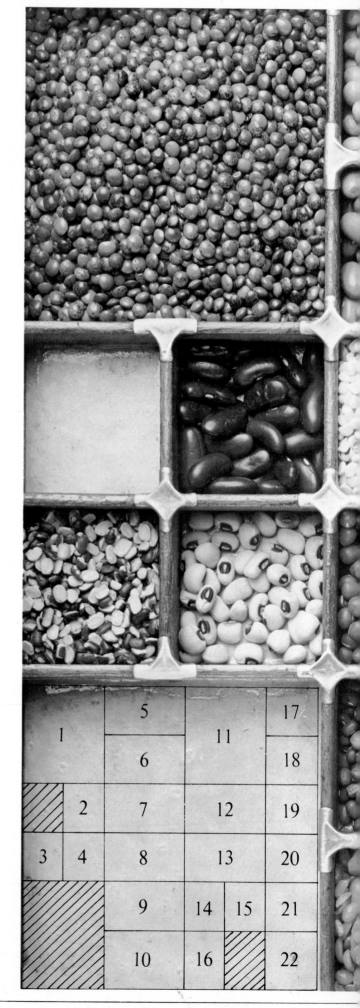

1. Brown lentils
2. Red kidney beans
3. Split kalay
4. Black eye peas
5. Soya beans
6. Dutch brown beans
7. Blanched lentils
8. Azuki
9. Mung
10. Yellow split peas
11. Sugar beans
12. Black beans
13. Red lentils
14. Kalay
15. Borlotti
16. Butter (dried Lima) beans
17. Chick peas
18. Yellow split peas
19. Haricots (Canellini)
20. Green lentils
21. Lupini
22. Dried green peas

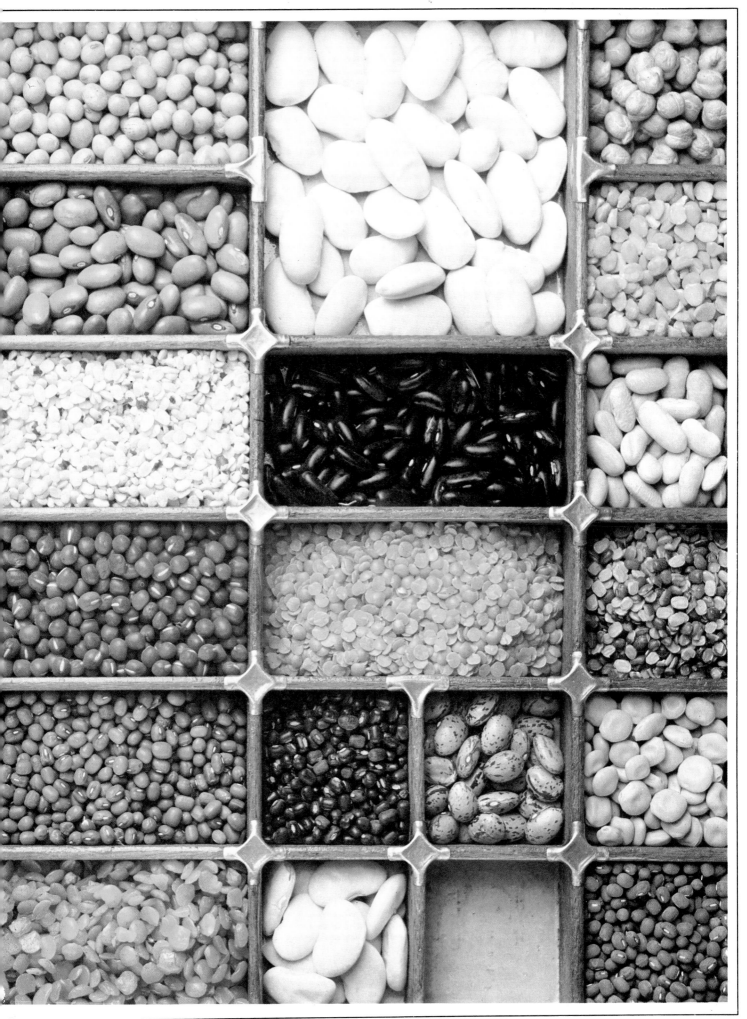

molasses

Molasses has been described as a crude mixture of sugars and minerals, and because of this natural 'crudeness' many people feel it can be a useful diet addition. However, most nutritionists say that the vitamins and minerals in molasses are readily available in other foods in sufficient quantities to provide good nutrition, and there is, therefore, no need to take molasses as a dietary supplement. On the other hand, where there is a choice between sugar and molasses—as in cooking—molasses is certainly better food-value.

Refined white sugar is extraordinarily high in carbohydrates—105 grams of sugar contains 100 grams of carbohydrates. But it contains very little else. Molasses is rich in magnesium, calcium, sodium and potassium salts, copper and the vitamins of the B group. Molasses alone will not supply sufficient quantities of these nutrients without the contribution of other foods, but it can certainly help and it is infinitely preferable to 'pure' sugar.

Jaggery or 'gur'

Indian cooks generally use jaggery whenever a sweetener is required. It is similar to molasses, can be obtained from health-food and oriental or speciality stores and is made from the juice of either the sugar cane or the palm. Sweeter than molasses, its colour ranges from dark brown to cream. In India it is used both as a food and as a medicine for rheumatism and intestinal disorders.

Minerals and vitamins in molasses	
Minerals	mg. per 100 grams
Sodium	96.0
Potassium	147
Calcium	497
Magnesium	144
Iron	9.17
Phosphorous	30.6
Sulphur	68.5
Chlorine	815
Vitamins	mg. per 100 grams
B1 (thiamine)	0.89
B2 (riboflavin)	0.3
Niacin (nicotinic acid)	4.7
Pantothenic acid	4.29
Choline	6.44

Coffee shake

This drink is almost a meal in itself. It is rich in both protein and vitamins, and if you are having it as a snack lunch you could add an egg yolk.
Preparation time: *5 minutes*
S E R V E S 1

6 fl. oz. [¾ cup] milk
½ teaspoon dried skim milk powder
1 teaspoon brewer's yeast powder
1 teaspoon molasses
1 teaspoon clear honey
1 teaspoon instant decaffeinated coffee powder
To garnish:
nutmeg

Pour the milk into the blender container. Add all the remaining ingredients and blend at full speed for 2 minutes. If you do not have a blender, place in a fairly deep bowl and whisk for 3 minutes. Pour into a glass.
Grate a little nutmeg on the surface before serving.

Molasses and chocolate cooler

Molasses blends well with milk, spices and chocolate to make this delicious and highly nutritious drink. Use it as a hot-weather treat for children or as a mid-morning pick-me-up for yourself.
Preparation time: *40 minutes*
S E R V E S 1

½ tablespoon molasses
a pinch of ground ginger
¼ teaspoon ground cinnamon
2 tablespoons hot water
6 fl. oz. [¾ cup] milk, ice cold
½ teaspoon grated plain [semi-sweet] chocolate
1 scoop vanilla ice-cream (optional)

Stir the molasses and spices into the hot water until they are well-mixed. Allow to cool.
Add the milk, sprinkle with the grated chocolate and, if liked, top with a scoop of ice-cream.

Molasses meringue

This is a spectacular dessert for special occasions when you want to impress guests with something different. The rich taste of the molasses blends well with the strawberry jam.

As this dish is very filling serve it after a fairly simple main course.
Preparation and cooking time:
45 minutes
S E R V E S 4

8 fl. oz. [1 cup] milk
½ tablespoon molasses
2 oz. fresh wholemeal [1 cup wholewheat] breadcrumbs
2 egg yolks
3 tablespoons strawberry jam (home-made if possible)
For the meringue topping:
2 egg whites
1 tablespoon castor [fine] sugar
½ tablespoon molasses

Heat the oven to 375°F (Gas Mark 5, 190°C).
Warm the milk and dissolve the molasses in it. Place the breadcrumbs in a basin, pour in the milk mixture and allow to cool slightly. Beat the egg yolks into the breadcrumb mixture.
Transfer to a greased pie dish and allow to stand for 20 minutes. Then bake in the oven for 15-20 minutes or until firm.
Remove from the oven and allow to cool slightly. Spread with strawberry jam.
Raise the oven heat to 450°F (Gas Mark 8, 230°C).
Beat the egg whites until stiff but not dry, add castor sugar and beat again until smooth. Beat in the molasses. Spread this meringue mixture over the jam and place in the oven for 5 minutes, until top is firm and crisp.
Serve at once.

Tasting as good as a milk shake, Molasses and Chocolate Cooler is a favourite with children.

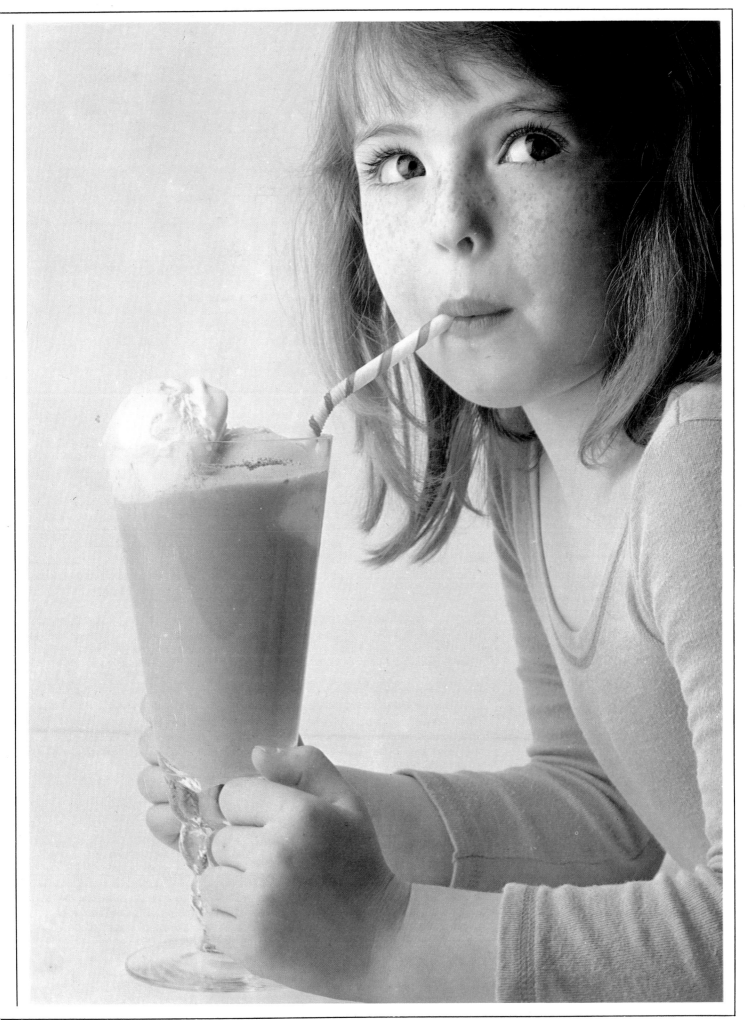

kelp-
for minerals

Kelp is a type of seaweed found on rocky ocean beds and shores. There are about 900 different species, but kelp tablets are made from the common *fucus vesiculosus*, a brownish seaweed with flat, fan-like fronds and air bubbles which children love to 'pop'.

Kelp and minerals

The real nutritional value of kelp lies in the mineral salts it contains. Trace quantities of these minerals are vital to good health, but refining and processing of other foods in which they are present often destroys them and although some are replaced at the end of the manufacturing process others are not. The importance of minerals in body metabolism is only just being fully explored, and until you know the exact amounts you need it makes sense to get your fair share or more. So, what do you get from kelp? Here is a full list: aluminium, barium, calcium, chromium, copper, iodine, lead, magnesium, manganese, potassium, silicon, silver, sodium, strontium, tin, titanium, vanadium, zinc.

Iodine is essential for the correct functioning of the thyroid gland. Copper helps the body to utilize vitamin C. Magnesium helps to keep bones and teeth strong, hair shiny and nails in good health. Manganese is vital for the nervous system and sexual drive. And so the list goes on.

The sensible, diet-conscious person would find many of these things in other foods. Green vegetables, for example, contain magnesium; liver and kidney contain manganese and copper, and seafoods are all rich sources of iodine. But these good foods are not eaten in enough quantities to ensure adequate mineral supplies. Kelp tablets can, therefore, be of great use, particularly to people who eat a lot of expensive foods—cakes, biscuits, sweets, alcohol—which contribute very little in the way of nutritional value.

Kelp as a food

Seaweed was once a common and popular addition to the diet of people living near the sea, and was eaten raw or cooked. But the idea of cooking and eating seaweed is not now to everyone's taste. The Japanese lead in the consumption of kelp, and they export to Tai Wan, Hong Kong and Singapore. The kelp is 'farmed' along the Japanese coastline. It takes about two years to mature after being sown on rocks in the sea. It is then harvested, dried and stored to be re-constructed in salted water when needed.

To Western palates kelp often seems leathery and waxy in taste, although somehow not so bad when chopped finely and added to Chinese or Japanese dishes. Consequently the most usual way of including kelp in a Western diet is to take it in tablet form or to add the dried powder to soups or stews. And it is worth remembering that a heaped teaspoon of kelp powder will make a pint of jelly which sets very quickly and is virtually tasteless, so you can use it instead of gelatine. Add fruit or vegetable juice flavouring to it.

The recommended daily dosage of kelp is one 5-grain tablet a day, or two if your nails are splitting and you have an overall feeling of lowered vitality.

Carrot and celery cocktail

This cocktail is rich in essential vitamins and minerals.
Preparation time: *5 minutes*
SERVES 1

2 celery stalks
4-5 sprigs parsley
1 large carrot
4 fl. oz. [½ cup] pure apple juice (bottled)
a pinch of kelp powder

Wash the celery and parsley and scrape the carrot. Cut them into small pieces, place in a blender container with just enough water to make the machine run smoothly.

Blend for 2 minutes at medium speed. *Strain* through a sieve, pressing out all the juice. Mix this vegetable juice with the apple juice and season to taste with kelp.

Hot cheese herbed scones [biscuits]

These make a very good accompaniment to a soup and salad lunch.
Preparation and cooking time: *30 minutes*
SERVES 4

8 oz. wholewheat [2 cups wholemeal] flour
2 teaspoons baking powder
¼ teaspoon sea salt

a pinch of kelp powder
2 tablespoons margarine
4 tablespoons grated cheese
½ teaspoon dried marjoram
2 tablespoons buttermilk *or* sour milk

Heat the oven to 425°F (Gas Mark 7, 220°C).
Sift together the flour, baking powder, salt and kelp, and return to the bowl any bran left in the sieve.
Rub in the margarine, stir in the cheese and marjoram and mix to a dough with the buttermilk or sour milk. (A little more liquid may be added if necessary.)
Form into a round ¾-inch thick and cut into 4 pieces. Place on a greased baking sheet and bake for 10-12 minutes. Serve with hot butter.

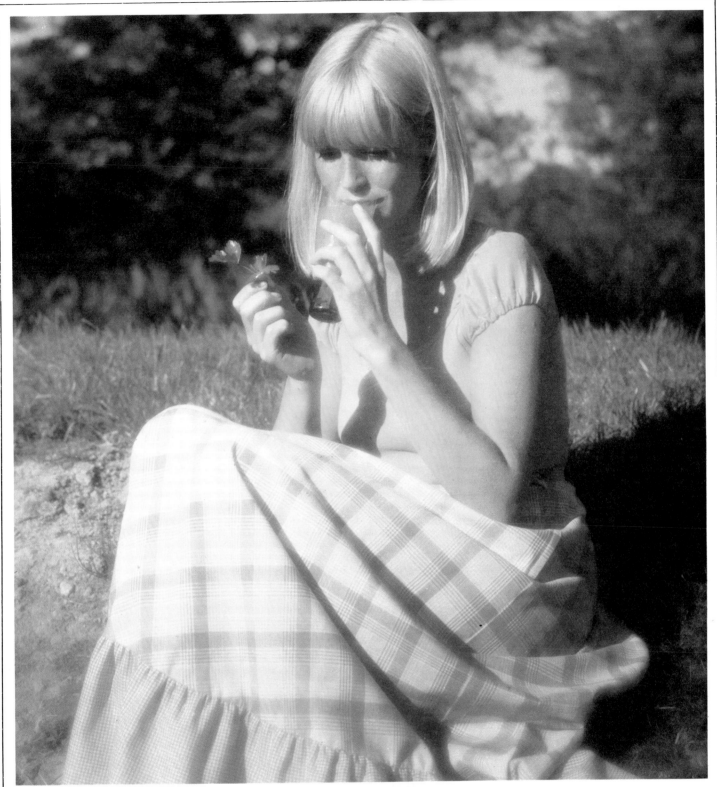

Onion lentil soup

Home-made soups are comforting on a cold day. This one has the extra protein of lentils and the minerals from powdered kelp.
Preparation and cooking time:
45 minutes
S E R V E S 4

12 oz. onions
8 oz. potatoes
2 tablespoons butter

2 tablespoons lentils
2 pints [5 cups] chicken stock
1 teaspoon kelp, or to taste
To serve:
parsley, chopped
grated cheese
fried croûtons or toast triangles

Peel and roughly chop the onions and potatoes. Melt the butter in a heavy pan and cook the vegetables, covered, over low heat until softened.
Meanwhile, grind the lentils to a fine powder in grinder or blender.

Carrot and Celery Cocktail makes a refreshingly different drink.

Add the lentils and stock to the softened vegetables, bring to the boil and simmer for 15 minutes. Cool slightly, pour into a blender or food mill and reduce to a smooth purée. *Return* to the pan, add a little more stock or milk if necessary, together with the seasoning of kelp powder. Bring back to boiling point, garnish with parsley and serve with cheese and croûtons or toast triangles.

apple cider vinegar

The minerals contained in apple cider vinegar are potassium, phosphorus, chlorine, sodium, magnesium, iron, fluorine and silicon—plus 'trace' amounts of several others. In the folk medicine lore of the hills of Vermont in America the potassium in apple cider vinegar is supposed to have bacteria-killing powers.

According to Doctor D. C. Jarvis, author of a best-selling book on the subject, bacteria take moisture from the body cells. But body cells contain potassium and this tends to draw moisture from bacteria. The constant fight between the body cells and the bacteria can, therefore, be tipped in favour of the body cells by taking potassium-rich foods—fruit, edible leaves, roots,

berries and apple cider vinegar. And the vinegar, Doctor Jarvis claims, is not only a good source of potassium but will also kill any bacteria lurking in the digestive tract.

Quite apart from its possible anti-bacteria powers and medicinal claims the minerals it contains make apple cider vinegar a good diet supplement. The usual recommended dose is two teaspoons mixed into a glass of water and taken once a day.

Remedies

Here is a list of some of the medicinal uses of apple cider vinegar. These cannot be vouched for, but none of them will do you any harm.

As a pick-me-up mix 2 teaspoons of

apple cider vinegar and 2 teaspoons of honey in a glass of warm water and take it whenever you feel low.

For fatigue take the following: mix three teaspoons of apple cider vinegar to one cup of honey. Take two teaspoons before meals and before going to bed.

For headaches put equal parts of apple cider vinegar and water into a saucepan. Bring to the boil and inhale the vapour.

Stomach upsets and mild food poisoning may be helped by taking 1 teaspoon of apple cider vinegar every few minutes until the symptoms are eased. As a preventive measure, drink 2 teaspoons of apple cider vinegar in a glass of water before eating.

French dressing

This is the classic recipe except that apple cider vinegar is substituted for the usual wine vinegar. You can make it up in advance—in larger quantities if you like—as it keeps well in the refrigerator.
Preparation time: *5 minutes*
M A K E S 1½ fluid ounces

¼ teaspoon sea salt
a pinch of freshly ground black
   pepper
¼ teaspoon dry mustard
1 tablespoon apple cider vinegar
2 tablespoons olive oil

Place all the ingredients in a screw-top jar and shake well. Use at once or store and re-shake before serving.

Mayonnaise

This is a fool-proof method of making a delicious mayonnaise which is in no danger of curdling.
Preparation and cooking time:
15 minutes, plus cooling time
M A K E S 1 pint [2½ cups]

1 tablespoon cornflour [cornstarch]
1 teaspoon mustard
5 fl. oz. [⅝ cup] skimmed milk
16 fl. oz. [2 cups] apple cider
   vinegar
2 egg yolks

Mix the cornflour [cornstarch] and mustard to a smooth cream with a little of the milk. Add the remainder of the milk and the vinegar. Stir in the egg yolks. Pour the mixture into a thick-bottomed saucepan, or a double saucepan if you have one, and heat gently stirring all the time until it thickens. Do not let it boil.
Allow to cool before serving.

Mousseline dressing

This is an attractive pink dressing to serve with fish dishes or a party salad platter. The tabasco gives a piquant flavour.
Preparation time: *5 minutes*
M A K E S 11 fluid ounces

5 fl. oz. double [⅝ cup heavy]
   cream
5 fl. oz. [⅝ cup] home-made
   mayonnaise* (recipe above)
1 teaspoon chopped fresh chives
1 teaspoon grated lemon zest
freshly ground black pepper
1 tablespoon tomato purée
1 tablespoon lemon juice
tabasco sauce

Fold the cream into the mayonnaise, combining well.
Add the chives, lemon zest and a little pepper. Then add tomato purée, lemon juice and a dash of tabasco to taste.

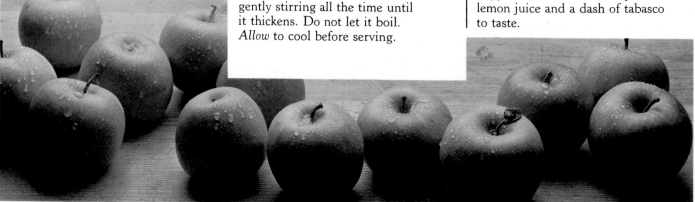

honey-energy food

Because it is easy to digest, honey is a good food for the very young and the elderly. There are many stories of exceptional longevity apparently caused by taking honey every day. And many athletes find it a good source of 'instant' energy.

How honey is made

Honey is nature's own manufactured food; harvested, processed and packed by bees. Bees are industrious little creatures. They have to be, because it takes about ten thousand flights—average length about two miles—for bees to bring a pound of nectar back to the hive. And nectar loses half its weight in evaporation!

The bee settles on a flower and sucks in the nectar. This passes into its honey sac and is mixed with acid secretions. Back at the hive the bee drops the nectar into honey 'houses'. (The biggest hive ever found was perched at the top of a giant eucalyptus tree in the Australian bush, it was 36 feet high, 21 feet across and weighed a ton.) From the 'houses' the nectar goes into honey vats and finally into the hexagonal cells of the wax honeycomb. The cells themselves are a remarkable achievement: accurate to within a thousandth of an inch, always identical and able to withstand temperatures of up to 140°F (60°C).

The flavour and texture of individual types of honey depends on the source of the nectar. Clover, heather, apple blossom and orange blossom are all popular kinds.

What honey contains

Honey contains three varieties of sugar: fructose, glucose and sucrose. The first, fructose, is a white crystalline substance which melts at 187°F (86°C). (It is sometimes called grape sugar as it is also found in grapes.) Glucose is the simplest of sugars. It is found in the blood of live animals (including humans), fruit and plant juices. Sucrose is the same as cane or beet sugar, and is a combination of fructose and glucose.

So, if honey is mainly a composition of three sugars, why is it reputed to have 'magical' properties? The known 'extras' in honey are the minerals—calcium, iron, phosphates, magnesium and iodine—and traces of at least six vitamins—B1, B2, C, pantothenic acid, pyridoxine and niacin. Then there are the 'undetermined residues' — resins, gums, etc.

Because it contains these important extras, honey is certainly a good choice as a sweetening ingredient in cooking. It is versatile, too. Honey vinegar and mead are two important by-products. Honey vinegar makes quite a good salad dressing. (You can make it yourself by boiling five parts of water to one of honey in an earthenware dish, adding a little yeast and leaving it to ferment for a few weeks in a warm room.)

Honey biscuits [cookies]

These biscuits [cookies] taste marvellous with mid-morning coffee or tea.
Preparation and cooking time:
45 minutes
MAKES 20 biscuits [cookies]

2½ oz. [5 tablespoons] **butter**
2 tablespoons **sugar**
2 tablespoons **honey**
6 oz. [1½ cups] **flour, sifted**
1½ teaspoons **baking powder**
1 teaspoon **cinnamon**
a pinch of **salt**

Heat the oven to 350°F (Gas Mark 4, 180°C).
Cream together butter and sugar. Add honey and work into the mixture with the flour, baking powder, cinnamon and salt. Roll out on a floured board to a ¾-inch thickness.
Cut into 40 small rounds, place on a greased baking sheet and bake for 10 minutes.
Allow to cool then sandwich rounds together in pairs, putting a little honey between each pair.
Serve-immediately.

Honey raisin pudding

This delicious steamed pudding includes energy-giving honey and dried fruits plus extra bran, so it is very good for you.
Preparation and cooking time:
1¼ hours
SERVES 4-6

4 oz. [½ cup] **margarine**
4 oz. [¾ cup] **soft brown sugar**
2 **eggs**
3 oz. [¾ cup] **flour**
½ teaspoon **baking powder**
1 oz. [¼ cup] **bran**
4 tablespoons **raisins**
4 tablespoons **clear honey**

Cream together margarine and sugar. Beat in the eggs one at a time, adding a little flour between additions. Fold in the remaining flour, the baking powder and bran. Stir in the raisins.
Grease a large pudding basin, spoon in the honey and top with the pudding mixture so that the basin is not more than two-thirds full. Cover with foil and steam for 1 hour.
Turn out and serve with extra honey and yogurt, or cream if preferred.

Mead

Although you have to wait a long time before drinking your mead the results are well worth while.
MAKES 1 gallon

3 lb. **honey**
the grated zest of 1 lemon
1 gallon cold **water**
2 **egg whites**
¼ oz. **fresh yeast**

Put the honey and grated lemon zest into a large saucepan or preserving pan and add the water. Beat the whites of the eggs until frothy and add to the pan. Place it over a low heat and stir as the mixture comes to the boil. Simmer gently for 1 hour.
Pour the liquid into a large bowl and leave until lukewarm. Stir in the yeast. Cover and leave in a warm place for three days, stirring daily.
Strain the liquid through muslin and bottle. Put the corks in loosely and take care they do not work out as the mead ferments. Gradually push them in tighter as fermentation slows down.
Store the bottles in a cold place for at least a year before drinking.

Muesli

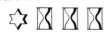

This is one version of the popular Swiss breakfast food.
Preparation time:
10 minutes, plus 12 hours soaking time for oats
S E R V E S 1

1 tablespoon oat flakes or oatmeal
3 tablespoons water
1 tablespoon lemon juice
1 cup milk, mixed with 1
   tablespoon honey
1 large apple
1 tablespoon grated nuts

Soak the oats or oatmeal in the water for about 12 hours, or overnight.
Mix together the lemon juice and the milk and honey mixture and pour this over the oats. Wash the apple, remove stalk and core and grate into the mixture. Top with grated nuts and serve at once.

Sesame honey scones
[biscuits]

The tiny sesame seed is rich in proteins, vitamins and minerals.
Preparation and cooking time:
30 minutes
S E R V E S 4

8 oz. [2 cups] **flour**
2 teaspoons **baking powder**
½ teaspoon **sea salt**
2 tablespoons **margarine**
4 tablespoons **wheat germ**
2 tablespoons **soft brown sugar**
1 tablespoon **sesame seeds**
2 tablespoons **clear honey**
3 fl. oz. [⅜ cup] **buttermilk** *or*
   sour milk

Heat the oven to 425°F (Gas Mark 7, 220°C).
Sift the flour with the baking powder and salt. Rub in the margarine, then stir in the wheat germ, sugar and half the sesame seeds.
Stir in the honey and buttermilk or sour milk and mix to a dough.
Form into a round ¾-inch thick and cut into 4 pieces. Scatter the rest of the sesame seeds over the top. Bake on a greased sheet for 10-15 minutes. Cool on a wire tray. Serve split in half and spread with butter

Honey Biscuits [cookies] and Sesame Honey Scones [biscuits] are ideal for an energy-giving mid-morning break.

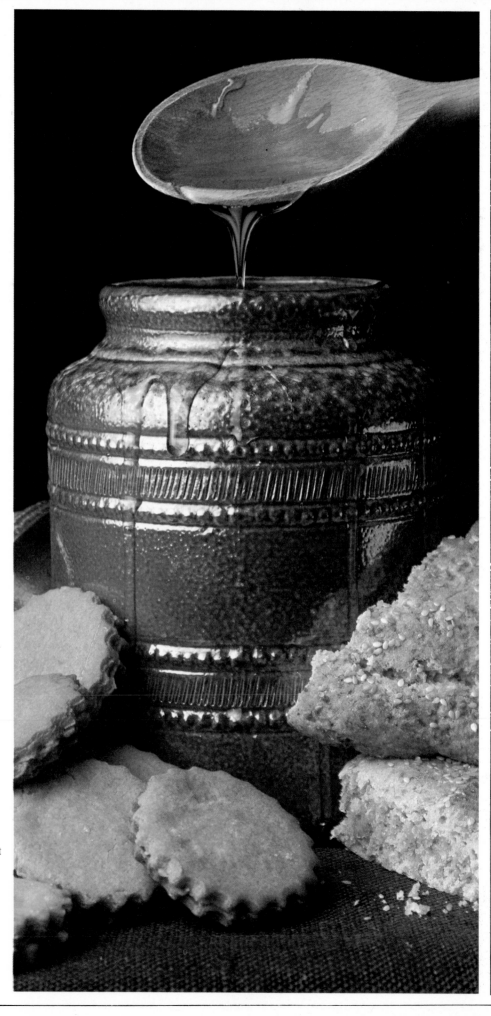

yeast & wheat germ-bread

Bread is no longer, nutritionally-speaking, considered to be 'the staff of life'. In affluent Western society we eat a variety of foods which contribute to a balanced diet, so most of us do not rely on bread as the main source of nutrients. It would, however, be wrong to play down the importance of bread as a top contributor to efficient body metabolism, particularly as most people eat some bread every day—something which cannot be said of any other food.

However, not all breads are equally good for you. Wholemeal [wholewheat] bread is best (see flour chart) because not only does it contain the vitamin B found in yeast but it also gives you the added goodness of wheat germ. And it tastes better, too, as you will discover when you try some of the recipes below.

Yeast—rich source of vitamin B

'Yeast' is the group name given to microscopic organisms or fungi which are carried from the soil to plants by the wind or by insects. Yeast is a living thing. When it is 'fed' on a sugar solution the cells which make up the organism divide and re-divide very rapidly producing alcohol and carbon dioxide. This process is called fermentation.

In the preparation of alcoholic drinks the sugar solution usually consists of fruit, grain or molasses together with water; the yeast is added and the alcohol which results is retained, while the carbon dioxide is given off. In bread-making, however, the reverse occurs. The yeast action traps the 'bubbles' of carbon dioxide in the bread—making it rise—and the alcohol is released.

The history of yeast

Yeast has been used as a fermentation agent for many centuries—there is even a reference to it as a cure for constipation in a scroll dating from the Egyptian 18th Dynasty (1567—1320 BC). Until comparatively recently, however, yeast was simply accepted, it was not understood.

Wild yeast was used for making wines and breads up until the 1870s then Emil Christian Hansen, a Danish scientist, discovered that it was possible to cultivate a pure strain of yeast. After that it was found that the live yeast fungi could be dried and later reconstituted with water without losing its 'living' properties. (Until then, housewives had been using liquid yeast bought from the local bakery, and this was messy and difficult to store.) In the 1930s when vitamin B was discovered, yeast turned out to be one of its best sources.

Vitamin value

The types of yeast commonly used today are *Torula utilis*, food yeast, and *Saccharomyces cerevisiae*, brewer's and baker's yeast. As a food supplement brewer's yeast is richest in protein containing all 15 members of the valuable B complex. It is a superb source of riboflavin and nicotinic acid and is second only to peanuts as a source of thiamine. Riboflavin is particularly important for normal growth of skin, nails and hair, and trichologists often recommend yeast tablets for hair in poor condition.

The importance of yeast depends upon what else you eat. Other rich sources of vitamin B exist, but where these are excluded from the diet because of personal taste or, as in some countries, poverty, then yeast can be a superb food supplement. Take it dried and sprinkled on milk, soups, salads and casserole dishes or in tablet form. And use it in home-made bread.

Wheat germ—the most valuable part of grain

Wheat germ is a rich source of vitamins A and E and of those of the B complex, and so it can be a very valuable part of your diet. (See pages 70-71 for the importance of these vitamins.) The wheat germ contains more than 50 per cent of all the vitamins found in the grain and is the only part that contains vitamin A.

To get a clear picture of exactly what wheat germ is, imagine a grain of wheat cut in half. There are three main parts: the bran, which makes up about 13-15 per cent of the grain, is a protective outer covering, difficult to digest for some people but a valuable source of roughage; the endosperm, which makes up about 82-86 per cent of the grain, consists mainly of starch and helps the grain to germinate and the seedling to develop; and, finally, the germ. This is a small part of the whole—only about 2.2-2.9 per cent. It is straw-coloured, a rich source of vitamin A, B and E and alive.

Unfortunately the general preference for white, light, easily-digestible bread means taking away this vitamin-rich wheat germ and bran—this is what gives wholemeal [wholewheat] bread its rough, nutty taste.

Vitamin value

As a dietary supplement, wheat germ can play an important part in maintaining good health—especially for the many people whose basic diet is fairly low in vitamins B and E. (The vitamin A contained in wheat germ is certainly of value but the quantity is less than half that present in a comparable amount of the fish liver oils.) It makes sense to get your fair share of these two valuable vitamins. A good way of doing so is either to eat wholemeal [wholewheat] bread or use wheat germ in cooking or sprinkled on food. Wheat germ gives a pleasantly nutty flavour and crunchy texture to foods, especially when used on cereals or stirred into fruit and vegetable juices. You could try it, too, cooked just as if it were a form of porridge and served with honey and milk as a breakfast food. If, however, you honestly dislike the taste, then you can take wheat germ oil in capsule form.

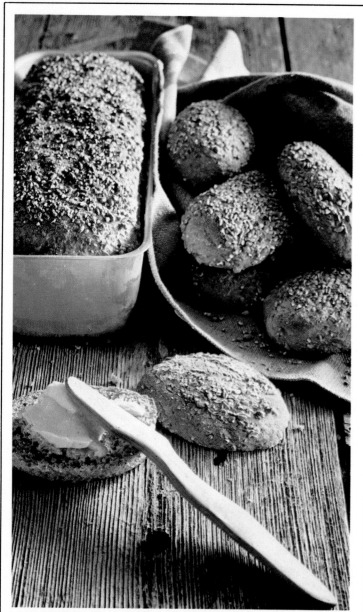

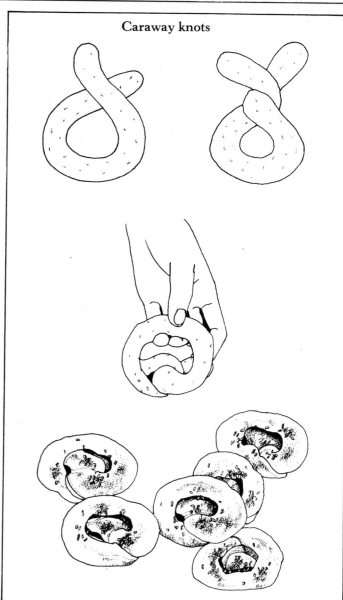

Caraway knots

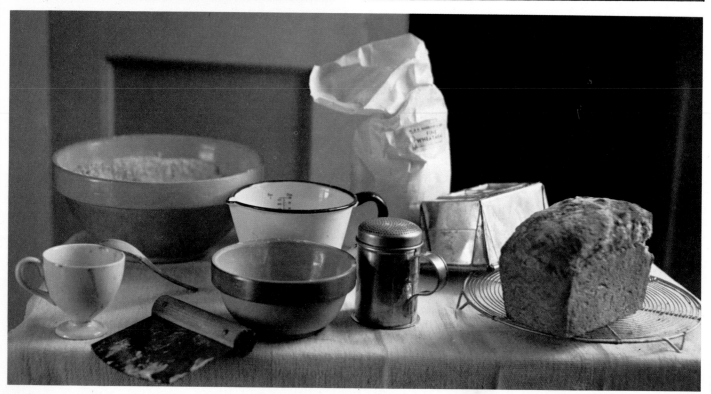

Baps

These soft, white, breakfast rolls are best served hot from the oven with lots of butter.
Preparation and cooking time:
$3\frac{1}{2}$ hours
MAKES 8 baps

$\frac{1}{2}$ oz. fresh yeast
$\frac{1}{2}$ teaspoon sugar
5 fl. oz. [$\frac{5}{8}$ cup] **lukewarm water**
5 fl. oz. [$\frac{5}{8}$ cup] **plus 2 tablespoons milk**
2 oz. [$\frac{1}{4}$ cup] **plus 1 teaspoon butter** *or* **margarine**
1 lb. [4 cups] **plus 1 tablespoon flour**
$\frac{1}{2}$ teaspoon sea salt

Crumble the yeast into a small mixing bowl and mash in the sugar with a kitchen fork. Add 2 tablespoons of the lukewarm water and cream the yeast and water together. Set the bowl aside in a warm, draught-free place for 15 to 20 minutes or until the yeast mixture has risen and is puffed up and frothy.
Meanwhile, in a small saucepan, scald 5 fluid ounces [$\frac{5}{8}$ cup] of the milk over moderate heat. Do this by bringing it to just under boiling point. Remove the pan from the heat and add 2 ounces [$\frac{1}{4}$ cup] of the butter or margarine. Set the pan aside to allow the milk to cool to lukewarm.
Sift the 1 pound [4 cups] of flour and the salt into a large, warmed mixing bowl. Make a well in the centre of the flour and add the yeast and milk mixture and the remaining water. Using your fingers or a spatula, gradually draw the flour into the liquid. Continue mixing until all the flour is incorporated and the dough comes away from the sides of the bowl.
Turn the dough out onto a lightly floured surface and knead it for 10 minutes, reflouring the surface if the dough becomes sticky. It should be smooth and elastic.
Rinse, thoroughly dry and lightly grease the large mixing bowl. Form the dough into a ball and return it to the bowl. Cover the bowl with a clean cloth and set it aside in a warm, draught-free place for 1 to $1\frac{1}{2}$ hours or until the dough has risen and doubled in bulk.
Lightly grease a large baking sheet with the teaspoon of butter or margarine and coat it with the tablespoon of flour. Set aside.
Turn the risen dough out onto a lightly floured surface and knead it for 5 minutes. Divide the dough into eight equal pieces and pat and roll each piece into an oval shape.
Flatten each oval and place it on the prepared baking sheet. Cover with a clean cloth and set aside in a warm, draught-free place for 30 minutes.
Heat the oven to 425°F (Gas Mark 7, 220°C).
Brush each bap with the remaining 2 tablespoons of milk and place the baking sheet in the oven. Bake the baps for 15-20 minutes or until they are golden brown.

Making your own bread is simpler than it sounds—and it is well worthwhile.

Caraway knots

These popular savoury knots are delicious served warm with butter.
Preparation and cooking time:
3 hours
MAKES 20 knots

$\frac{3}{4}$ oz. fresh yeast
1 tablespoon sugar
2 teaspoons lukewarm water
15 fl. oz. [$1\frac{7}{8}$ cups] **milk**
2 oz. [$\frac{1}{4}$ cup] **butter or margarine**
2 lb. [8 cups] **plus 1 tablespoon flour**
1 tablespoon sea salt
2 eggs
3 tablespoons caraway seeds
1 teaspoon vegetable oil

Crumble the yeast into a small mixing bowl and mash in 1 teaspoon of the sugar with a kitchen fork. Add the warm water and cream the yeast and water together. Set the bowl aside in a warm, draught-free place for 15 to 20 minutes or until the yeast mixture has risen and is puffed up and frothy.
Pour the milk into a small saucepan, place it over low heat, and bring it to just under boiling point. Remove the pan from the heat and add the butter or margarine. When the butter or margarine has melted, set the pan aside and leave the milk to cool to lukewarm.
Sift the 2 pounds [8 cups] of flour, the salt and the remaining sugar into a medium-sized mixing bowl. Make a well in the centre and pour in the yeast mixture and milk mixture. Add one of the eggs. Using a wooden spoon or your hands, gradually incorporate the flour into the liquid. Continue mixing until a smooth dough is formed.
Fold in 2 tablespoons of caraway seeds. Sprinkle the remaining flour over the dough. Cover the bowl with a cloth and put it in a warm, draught-free place to rise for 1 to $1\frac{1}{2}$ hours or until the dough has almost doubled in bulk.
Turn the risen dough out on to a lightly floured surface and knead it for about 5 minutes or until it is smooth.
Roll the dough into a 12-inch long roll and with a sharp knife slice it into 20 equal pieces. Roll one piece between your hands to make a thin rope about 14 inches long. Place the rope on a board and shape it into a loop with its ends crossed. Turn the ends of the rope over again to make a twist at the base of the loop. Spread the tips of the two ends apart, bring the loop over to them and pinch the tips to the loop. Do the same with each piece of dough. After all the knots have been formed, leave them to rest for 10 minutes.
Using a pastry brush, lightly grease two baking sheets with the oil. Set aside.
Fill a large saucepan two-thirds full of water. Bring the water to the boil over high heat. Lay 2 knots at a time in the water. The knots will sink to the bottom, and then rise to the surface of the water and will double in size.
With a slotted spoon, carefully transfer the knots from the water to the greased baking sheets. (If the knots have come untwisted, gently press them into their original shape.)
Leave the knots in a warm place for 15 minutes or until they are almost dry.
Heat the oven to 400°F (Gas Mark 6, 200°C).
Beat the remaining egg. Using a pastry brush, coat the knots with the beaten egg and sprinkle them with the rest of the caraway seeds. Place the knots in the oven and bake them for 15 to 20 minutes, or until they are golden brown.
Remove the knots from the oven and transfer them to a wire rack.
Serve warm.

One rise brown loaf

This loaf needs less rising time than most bread recipes, but it will not keep for as long as other breads. Eat it the day you bake it if possible.
Preparation and cooking time:
$1\frac{1}{2}$ hours

MAKES 1 x 2lb. loaf

½ teaspoon sugar
15 fl. oz. [1⅞ cups] tepid water
   (110°F, 43°C)
1 tablespoon dried yeast
12 oz. wholemeal
   [3 cups wholewheat] flour
12 oz. [3 cups] flour
2 teaspoons sea salt
2 teaspoons oil

Prepare the yeast liquid. Dissolve
the sugar in the warm water, sprinkle
in the yeast and leave for ten
minutes or until frothy.
Sift together the flours and salt,
and return to the bowl any bran left
in the sieve. Add the oil and work in
the yeast liquid to make a firm ball
of dough which comes away from the
sides of the bowl. Knead well on a
lightly floured surface for 5 minutes.
Heat the oven to 475°F (Gas Mark 8,
240°C).
Place the dough in a greased 2-pound
loaf tin, slip into a large oiled plastic
bag and leave to rise in a warm place
for about 1 hour or until doubled in
bulk. When sufficiently risen, the
dough should spring back when lightly
pressed.
Bake in oven for ten minutes then
reduce oven temperature to 425°F
(Gas Mark 7, 220°C) and bake for a
further 35 minutes, or until brown.
Cool on a wire tray.

Sour dough bread

⧖ ⧖ ⧖

This delicious bread is based upon
the Bavarian recipe, not the
American one. It will keep for a
week or more if stored in a bread
bin or crock.
Preparation and cooking time:
*4½ hours, plus 4 to 5 days for the
sour dough starter*
MAKES 2 x 2lb. loaves
   or 4 x 1lb. loaves

1 oz. fresh *or* dried yeast
¼ teaspoon sugar
1½ pints [3 cups] water, lukewarm
1½ lb. [6 cups] strong plain
   [all-purpose] flour *or* stoneground
   wholemeal [wholewheat] flour
1½ lb. [6 cups] stoneground rye
   flour
4 oz. [½ cup] cracked wheat
1½ tablespoons dark brown sugar
1½ tablespoons coarse rock salt
2 tablespoons vegetable oil
1½ tablespoons culinary malt
   (optional)

For the sour dough starter:
8 oz. strong plain
   [2 cups all-purpose] flour
8 oz. [2 cups] stoneground rye flour
4 oz. [½ cup] sugar
16 fl. oz. [2 cups] milk
For the glaze:
1 egg, beaten
2 teaspoons cold water

Put all the ingredients for the sour
dough starter into a large screw top
jar or container with a tight lid.
Mix it well with a fork. Screw on the
lid and leave it undisturbed at room
temperature for 4-5 days.
Grease loaf tins with butter and set
aside.
Crumble the yeast in a small bowl and
mash in ¼ teaspoon sugar with a
kitchen fork. Add 10 fluid ounces
[1¼ cups] of the water and mix
together. Set aside in a warm,
draught-free place for 15-20 minutes
or until the yeast has risen and is
puffed up and frothy.
Put the flours, cracked wheat, dark
brown sugar and salt into a very large
mixing bowl. Mix well together.
Add the vegetable oil, and culinary
malt if you are using it, to the
remaining water and mix together.
Make a well in the centre of the
flour mixture, pour in the yeast
mixture, the water, malt and oil
mixture and the sour dough starter.
Using your fingers or a spatula mix
well together until all the flour is
incorporated and the dough comes
away from the sides of the bowl.
Turn the dough on to a floured
surface and knead for about 5 minutes.
Rinse, thoroughly dry and lightly
grease the large mixing bowl. Shape
the dough into a ball and return it
to the bowl. Dust the top of the
dough with flour and cover the bowl
with a clean damp cloth. Set aside in
a warm, draught-free place and leave
to rise for 1½-2 hours or until the
dough has risen and almost doubled
in bulk.
Turn the dough out on to a floured
surface and knead again for 8-10
minutes. Using a sharp knife cut it
into required loaf sizes, put it into
the greased tins, cover with a damp
cloth and leave in a warm place to
rise again for another 1 to 1½ hours.
Heat the oven to 475°F (Gas Mark 9,
240°C).
Mix together the egg and water
glazing and paint the top of the
loaves with it.
Place tins in centre of oven and bake
for 10 minutes. Then lower oven
temperature to 425°F (Gas Mark 7,

220°C) put the bread on a lower shelf
and bake for another 30-40 minutes.
Remove the loaves from the oven, tip
them out and tap the undersides with
your knuckles. If the bread sounds
hollow like a drum it is cooked. If
not, return to the oven for a further
10 minutes.
Cool the loaves on a wire rack.

Wholemeal
[wholewheat] bread

⧖ ⧖ ⧖

This bread is simple to make at
home. It is fragrant and delicious
and retains all the goodness of
the wheat.
Preparation and cooking time:
3 hours
MAKES 2 x 1 lb. loaves

½ teaspoon sugar
15 fl. oz. [1⅞ cups] tepid water
   (110°F, 43°C)
1 tablespoon dried yeast
1½ lb. wholemeal [6 cups
   wholewheat] flour
½ tablespoon sea salt
2 teaspoons oil
1 tablespoon soft brown sugar

Prepare the yeast liquid. Dissolve
the sugar in the warm water, sprinkle
in the yeast and leave for 10 minutes
or until frothy.
Sift together the flour and salt, and
return to the bowl any residue left in
the sieve. Mix in oil and sugar. Work
in the yeast liquid to make a firm
ball of dough which comes away from
the sides of the bowl. Knead
thoroughly on a lightly floured
surface for about 10 minutes until
the dough is smooth and elastic.
Replace in bowl, cover with a large
greased plastic bag and leave in a
warm place for 1 hour or until risen
to double its bulk. The dough should
spring back when gently pressed.
Heat the oven to 475°F (Gas Mark 9,
240°C).
Turn out and knead well, flattening
with the knuckles to knock out air
bubbles. Place in 2 greased 1-pound
loaf tins, replace in loose plastic
bag leaving plenty of air space.
Leave to rise again for one hour or
until doubled in bulk.
Bake in the oven for 10 minutes then
lower the oven temperature to 425°F
(Gas Mark 7, 220°C), and bake for a
further 35 minutes. When done, the
loaf will shrink from the sides of the
tin, and will sound hollow if tapped.
Cool on wire tray.

flour-cakes

There is, as every cook knows, a tremendous difference between cakes you buy and those you make. Home-made cakes taste better for a start and you can make sure that they are nutritious as well, particularly if you choose your flour carefully.

Flour

Flours vary in composition. Broadly-speaking, they are defined by their rate of 'extraction'. This means the percentage of the whole grain (or wheat germ) which remains in the flour after milling. For example, wholemeal flours (wholewheat is another name for them) contain the *whole* of the cleaned wheat germ; brown or wheatmeal flours usually contain about 80 per cent to 90 per cent; white flours usually contain 70 to 72 per cent, and 'patent' flours (very white in colour) contain only 40-50 per cent of the germ. (If you can it is a good idea to use 80 per cent extraction flour when trying the recipes given here.)

Over, there is a table giving the comparative values of four different kinds of flour. (The dramatic increase in calcium in the whiter flours is due to calcium—in the form of chalk—being added during the refining processes.)

Banana nut bread

Tea breads are very simple to make and are always popular with a family.
Preparation and cooking time:
1 hour 15 minutes
MAKES 1 x 1 lb. loaf

2 oz. [¼ cup] **margarine**
2 oz. [⅓ cup] **soft brown sugar**
8 oz. [2 cups] **flour**
1 teaspoon **baking powder**
½ teaspoon **sea salt**
1 **egg**
2 ripe **bananas**
2 tablespoons **natural yogurt**
1 tablespoon **clear honey**
2 oz. [½ cup] **chopped walnuts**

Heat the oven to 350°F (Gas Mark 4, 180°C).
Cream the margarine with sugar.
Sift together the flour, baking powder and salt. Beat the egg into the fat with a little flour.
Mash the bananas, beat in with the yogurt and honey and gradually add to the egg mixture with the rest of the flour. Stir in the nuts.
Turn into a greased loaf tin and bake for 1¼-1½ hours, or until a skewer comes out clean when inserted. Cool on a wire tray and keep for 24 hours before cutting.

Ginger fruit cake

Sweetened with iron-rich black treacle [molasses], this cake is good for family snacks. Try it, too, with cheese for a picnic lunch.
Preparation and cooking time:
1¼ hours
MAKES 1 x 9-inch cake

4 oz. [½ cup] **margarine**
4 oz. [⅔ cup] **soft brown sugar**
8 oz. [2 cups] **flour**
1 teaspoon **baking powder**
1 teaspoon **ground ginger**
½ teaspoon **ground cinnamon**
½ teaspoon **sea salt**
2 **eggs**
5 fl. oz. **black treacle**
  [⅝ cup molasses]
3 fl. oz. [⅜ cup] **clear honey**
2 tablespoons **buttermilk** *or* sour milk
2 oz. [⅓ cup] **raisins**
2 oz. [⅓ cup] **cooking dates, chopped**
6-8 **almonds, blanched and shredded**

Heat the oven to 325°F, (Gas Mark 3, 170°C).
Cream together the margarine and sugar until fluffy.
Sift together the flour, baking powder, spices and salt. Beat the eggs into the fat, one at a time, adding half the flour. Beat the treacle, honey and buttermilk into the mixture and add the rest of the flour. Stir in the fruit.
Turn mixture into a greased 9-inch square cake tin and bake for 50-60 minutes, or until a skewer comes out clean. Sprinkle the almonds over the top after 40 minutes' cooking time.
Cool the cake on a wire tray and keep for 24 hours before cutting into squares.

Peanut coffee sandwich cake

This cake includes the extra nourishment of peanuts and soya flour, plus a delicious and unusual filling.
Preparation and cooking time:
50 minutes, plus cooling time
MAKES 1 x 8-inch cake

7 oz. [⅞ cup] **margarine**
7 oz. [1¼ cups] **soft brown sugar**
6 oz. [1½ cups] **flour**
1 teaspoon **baking powder**
4 tablespoons **soya flour**
3 large **eggs**
For the filling:
2 tablespoons **smooth peanut butter**
2 tablespoons **honey**
1 teaspoon **decaffeinated instant coffee powder**

Heat the oven to 350°F (Gas Mark 4, 180°C).
Cream the margarine and sugar thoroughly together.
Sift the flour with baking powder and soya. Beat eggs into the fat one at a time, adding a little flour between each one. Beat well, then fold in the remaining flour. Divide between two greased 8-inch sandwich tins.
Bake for 30 to 35 minutes, until the cake is well risen and when you insert a skewer it comes out clean. Cool on a wire rack.
To make the filling, beat the peanut butter and honey together. Dissolve the coffee in a teaspoon of boiling water and work into the honey mixture.

Spread this mixture on one layer of the cooled cake. Then place the second layer on top.

Sandringham tarts

Make these in small patty tins for mid-afternoon break. Alternatively, you can use the same mixture as the filling for an open tart for dessert.
Preparation and cooking time:
40 minutes
MAKES 12 tarts

For the pastry:
4 oz. [1 cup] flour
a pinch of sea salt
2 oz. [¼ cup] margarine
water
For the filling:
3 oz. [⅜ cup] margarine
3 oz. [½ cup] soft brown sugar
1 egg
3 oz. [¾ cup] ground unpolished rice
raspberry jam

Heat the oven to 400°F (Gas Mark 6, 200°C).
Sift together the flour and salt, rub in the margarine and add enough cold water to make a stiff dough. Roll out and use to line 12 patty tins.
To make the filling, cream together the margarine and sugar. Beat in the egg and the ground rice (unpolished rice may be ground at home in small quantities in a blender or grinder).
Place a teaspoonful of jam in the bottom of each tart. Divide the rice mixture between them and smooth over to cover the jam. Bake for 12-15 minutes. Cool on a wire rack.

Seed cake

This traditional caraway cake is always a favourite.
Preparation and cooking time:
2 hours
MAKES 1 x 1lb. cake

4 oz. [½ cup] butter
4 oz. castor [½ cup fine] sugar
2 eggs, beaten
8 oz. [2 cups] flour
2 teaspoons baking powder
2 teaspoons caraway seeds
4 tablespoons milk

Heat the oven to 350°F (Gas Mark 4, 180°C).
Cream together the butter and sugar

and add the eggs gradually, beating well.
Sift together the flour and baking powder and lightly fold into the mixture, adding the seeds and the milk as you go.
Put into a greased and floured cake tin and bake for about 1½ hours. The

cake is cooked when a skewer inserted into it comes out clean. Remove from the oven and cool on a wire rack.

The ingredients for Ginger Fruit Cake (recipe page 125) include raisins and dates, honey and molasses—all high in vitamins.

THE COMPARATIVE VALUES OF FLOUR

	Wholemeal	Brown	80% extraction	White enriched
Extraction Rate	100%	90%	80%	70%
Protein %	12.00	11.80	11.50	11.10
Fat %	2.49	1.90	1.40	1.16
Carbohydrate %	64.30	67.50	70.10	72.30
Calories per 100 grams	336.00	348.00	348.00	350.00
Calcium (mg. per 100 grams	30.00	148.00	145.00	142.00
Iron (mg. per 100 grams	3.50	2.70	1.70	1.70
Thiamine (mg. per 100 grams	0.40	0.33	0.24	0.24
Niacin (mg. per 100 grams	5.70	3.50	1.60	1.60

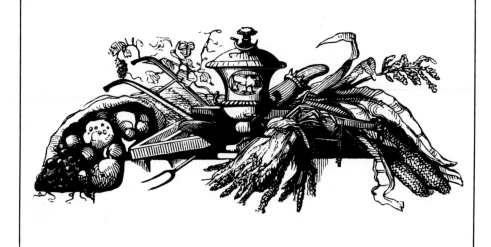

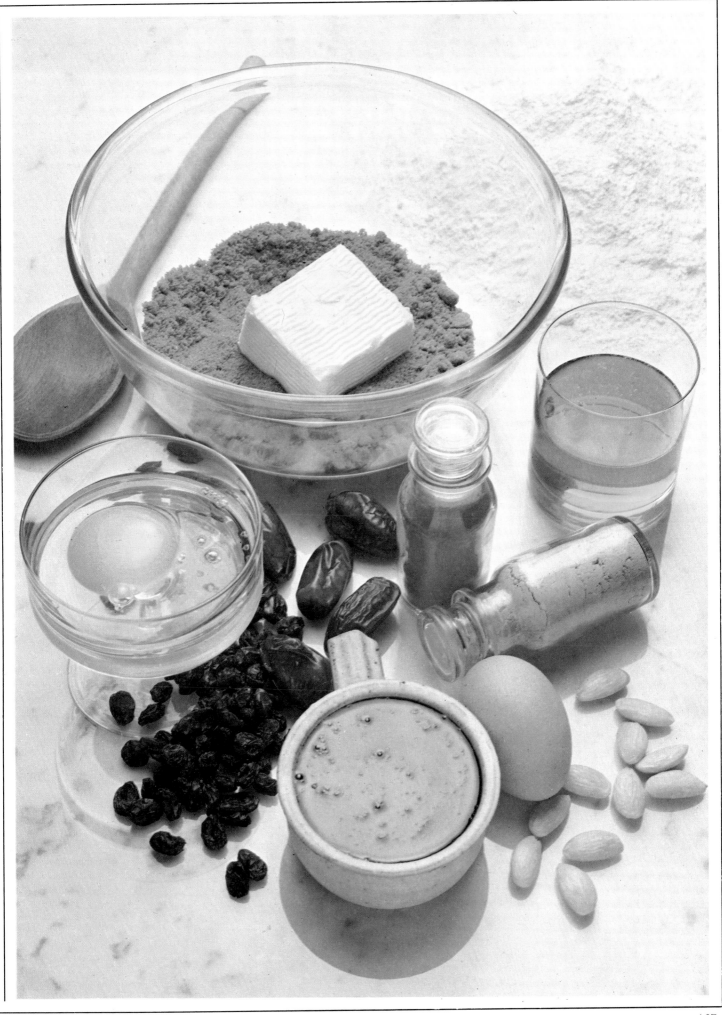

grow it

Even if you have a very small garden, it is possible to grow vegetables and herbs to add variety and nutritional value to everyday meals. And for flat-dwellers an indoor herb garden or a tiny salad plot in a window-box is a practical possibility. When space is limited the best plan is to decide which vegetables will give the best return. Choose quick-growing, easy-to-care-for plants which don't need a lot of space. Spinach, for example, is not only extremely nutritious: it is also practically self-perpetuating—the more you pick it the faster it grows. But you need to plant rows and rows of cabbages to feed a family throughout the winter. And, there is no point in planting rows of potatoes and turnips if you are not going to eat them.

The three top herbs for sheer usefulness are chives, parsley and mint. Grow them from seeds indoors or buy the plants in spring. When all danger of frost is past transfer them to a sheltered outside plot or window-box. Once these hardy plants take hold, they will spread fairly rapidly. Parsley is tops for food value and can be added to very many dishes. Use chives in soups, salads and sauces. Add mint to potatoes, vegetables and healthy drinks and use chopped fresh mint as a garnish.

Lettuces, spring onions [scallions], watercress and radishes need little space and are fairly easy to care for. Tomatoes can be grown indoors. Buy the plants in spring and rear them carefully in a box on a sunny window-sill. Mushrooms can be cultivated in any dark place—the cupboard under the stairs, the cellar or even the airing cupboard. Again they are so useful that growing them is well worth while. Give back the goodness which the plants extract from the soil by using compost (in the window-box, too). You can make a small compost heap with grass cuttings, leaves, twigs, vegetable peels and outer leaves, and newspapers and cardboard (paper was once a tree, after all). Spread this over the ground about a month before planting.

If space allows, and you have time to care for them, then soft fruits are a good idea. Strawberries, raspberries, blackcurrants, redcurrants and gooseberries are all delicious and useful for their food-value.

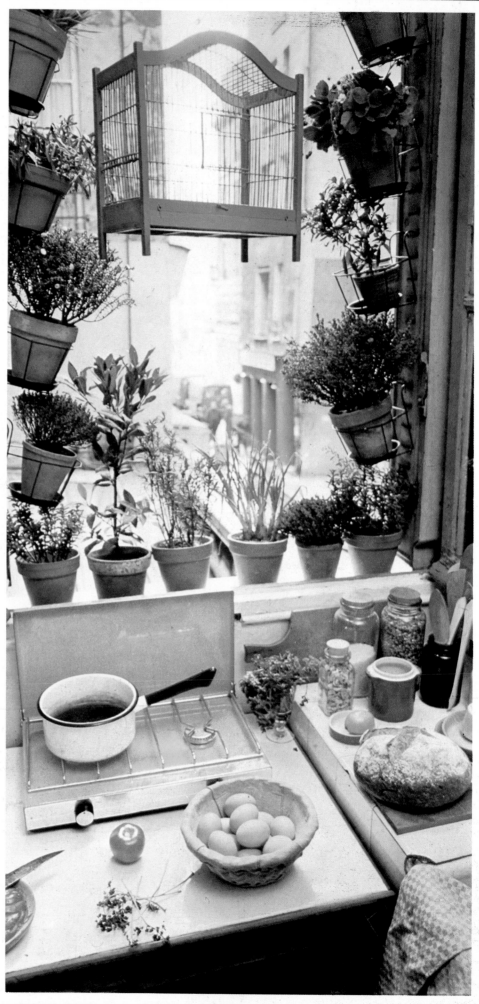